Alive
at 25

HOW I'M BEATING CYSTIC FIBROSIS

Andy Lipman

ℓLONGSTREET PRESS
Atlanta

Published by
LONGSTREET PRESS, INC.
2974 Hardman Court
Atlanta, GA 30305

Printed in the United States of America

1st printing 2001

Library of Congress Catalog Card Number: 2001091249

ISBN: 1-56352-681-6

Jacket and book design by Burtch Bennett Hunter
Edited by Ann Lovett

Alive
at 25

FOREWORD

"Hi Chipper." Those were all the words I needed to hear from the young man that was on the other end of my stare. He had me. Cystic Fibrosis had me.

The trip I took to the hospital that day changed the way that I look at CF, and more importantly, at my own life. I had always considered myself invincible. Being an athlete all my life, I had always assumed that my health would be with me. I had always assumed that I was indestructible. That changed that day.

I guess I just always took for granted what I had before me. I am a professional baseball player, a husband, and a dad. I have every dream that I ever imagined right in front of me. Having all of this, it was easy for me to take it for granted. Working with CF has made me appreciate the gifts that I have been given. I treasure my wife, my kids, and my health every day. I constantly think about my life in baseball, playing the game that I have grown to love and respect. Most importantly, however, I treasure my experiences in getting a chance to touch those with CF.

Sometimes we, as a society, want to see CF patients as beyond help, or with some sense of pity. I don't see CF patients in that way. CF patients don't see themselves in that way. I see CF patients enjoying life more completely than healthy individuals. I see CF patients doing things that others don't dare to do. In CF patients, I see a source of motivation and hope that things will get better. That things are never as bad as they seem.

I treasure my life in baseball each and every day. Borrowing a phrase from the great Joe DiMaggio, I try to play the game of baseball as if someone in the stands that day has never seen me play before. I believe that CF patients have lent this way of thinking to me. People like Andy Lipman live just as if someone had never seen him before. I am proud to be a part of the Bridges to a Cure Campaign and in the fight against this disease. I am proud to be writing this foreword to a book that tells people that life is there for the taking. And, I am proud to say that I know CF patients like Andy Lipman. Andy, we are all with you.

— Chipper Jones

5-Time All-Star Third Baseman for the Atlanta Braves

1999 National League Most Valuable Player

2001 Participant in the Bridges to a Cure Campaign for Cystic Fibrosis

INTRODUCTION

My own daughter, Alex, was born in 1971, and would be very near Andy Lipman's age had she not died when she was eight years old. But Andy, like Alex, has cystic fibrosis, and so I am very familiar with much of his story. It brings back many raw memories.

Andy has thrived, though. He hasn't beaten cystic fibrosis – we haven't quite figured how to do that *yet* – but in his own life, he certainly has gained the upper hand. And, in fact, so much of the courage of his story is bound up in the fact that Andy knows there is no easy victory for him, that he must keep fighting. That, I think, takes even more fortitude, to know that you must constantly keep at it, just to stay ahead of the game.

In some respects, though, Andy's story is not just about a young man with CF. The hurdles he has had to overcome, the setbacks, the anxieties, the embarrassments, the fears – these are some of the painful elements of growing up that almost all of us had to endure. But while we can identify some with Andy, it's also true that our own concerns then seem so very slight when we read about what Andy has suffered.

He does not spare himself, either. He lets us know how suffocating CF is, how it doesn't just smother the lungs but so much of your life – emotionally no less than physically. *Was the disease taking over again?* Andy cries out at one point. Growing up is hard enough to do without wondering if you will die.

But it is also the case that, in some respects, Andy's life mirrors the advances that have been found in the research battle against cystic fibrosis. Alex Deford, unfortunately, never really had a chance to overcome CF. She was my hero, a symbol of bravery, who was noble in her struggle against the disease. But she only fought the good fight. Alas, she could not win. Now, so many others – like Andy – are succeeding in that fight. "My goal is to finish what Alex started," Andy writes – and already he has run – not walked, but run – far along the path toward that goal. We can be sure that there will soon be a happy ending for all of the people who must suffer from cystic fibrosis.

Andy Lipman's story is inspirational. It is honest and painful, but ultimately one that is full of his joy and our admiration.

— Frank Deford

ABOUT CYSTIC FIBROSIS

(Facts provided by the CF Foundation)

Cystic fibrosis is a disease affecting approximately 30,000 children and adults in the United States. CF is not a virus or a cold. You cannot catch it from touching someone or through sexual intercourse. It is a genetic disorder, meaning that an individual must inherit a defective copy of the CF gene — one from each parent — to have cystic fibrosis. Each time two carriers conceive a child, there is a 25 percent chance that the child will have CF, a 50 percent chance that the child will be a carrier, and a 25 percent chance that the child will be a non-carrier. One in 31 Americans (one in 28 Caucasians) - more than 10 million people - is an unknowing, symptomless carrier of the defective gene.

CF (cystic fibrosis) causes the body to produce an abnormally thick, sticky mucus, due to the faulty transport of sodium and chloride within cells lining organs such as the lungs and pancreas, to their outer surfaces. One means of treatment, chest physical therapy, requires vigorous percussion (by using cupped hands) on the back and chest to dislodge the thick mucus from the lungs. Chest physical therapy usually requires the help of another person because of the difficulty in reaching certain parts of the body. These days, there is now a machine called "the vest" which enables a CFer to administer his or her own therapy. Antibiotics are also used to treat lung infections and are administered intravenously, via pills, and/or medicated vapors which are inhaled to open up clogged airways.

CF has a variety of symptoms. The most common are salty-tasting skin, persistent coughing, wheezing or pneumonia, and poor weight gain. The sweat test is the most common test to determine if a person has cystic fibrosis. This test measures the amount of salt in the sweat. A high salt level indicates that a person has CF. Most people are diagnosed with CF as infants.

Since the defective CF gene was discovered in 1989, the pace of CF research has greatly accelerated. In 1990, scientists successfully made copies of the normal gene, and then added them to CF cells in laboratory dishes, which corrected the defective cells. The next major step was achieved in early 1993 when the first experimental gene therapy treatment was given to a patient with CF. Researchers modified a common cold virus to act as a delivery vehicle - carrying the genes to the CF cells in the airways.

The median life expectancy for CF is 32 years, but this statistic is misleading. When I was born, the life expectancy was 12 years. And as a child, I read that I would not be breathing by my mid-twenties. It seems as more research has been done and more treatments have been discovered; these numbers have been on the rise. Though a cure is still roughly ten years away, the prognosis for someone with CF has greatly improved over the last several years.

Cystic fibrosis is a horrid disease. It kills hundreds of

people every year in the U.S. Many of these people are children who have yet to find love, go to college, or live a life without fear of what the next day will bring.

I have battled CF. My road has not been as tough as some others, but it hasn't been easy. And with CF it's not just the physical ailments, it's the emotional stress it puts on your life and the lives of those who care about you. I am not asking for your pity. When you read this book, you'll see that. What I'm asking for is your confidence. Your confidence that I will live a long life and that I will beat CF.

So when you read this book, I want you to see that CFers are like anybody else. We have our good days. We have our bad days. But we never stop fighting. When you finish reading *Alive at 25*, ask yourself one question. Have you achieved everything you've wanted from life? If the answer is "no," then go out there and beat your own "CF."

I have CF, but it will never have me!
— Andy Lipman

This book is dedicated to the girl of my dreams.
Looking forward to our next encounter . . .

C O N T E N T S

1	Stand and Deliver	1
2	What I'm Dealing With	9
3	Parental Guidance	13
4	Proving	25
5	My Kinship with Alex	31
6	My High School Tennis Days	39
7	Independence Day – My Machine Arrives	45
8	My Friend For Life	49
9	Growing Up in a Rush	55
10	Changing My Outlook	61
11	Rude Awakening	69
12	Why Me?	73
13	Fading Away	87
14	The Final Cry	93
15	The Basketball Game	99
16	The Recovery	111
17	Revenge	121
18	Oh, DIOS	125
19	The T-Shirt	135
20	The Bookmark	143
21	Dating: It's An Attitude	153
22	The Test	161
23	The Answer	167
24	Meeting Someone New: CF's No Longer Taboo	171
25	Athletics: My Way of Coping	179
26	The End of Isolation	187
27	More than a Name	195
28	Cemetery Meeting	203
29	A Wish for Wendy	213
30	Words to Live By	219

Alive
at 25

THE DREAM

I am sitting under a clothes rack. I think I am in the mall, but it could be some random department store. There are people moving on either side of me. I don't know any of them. None of them seem to notice me. I'm scared that I'm lost. I'm all alone. Then I see her.

A girl walks into the store and heads directly towards me. She has brown hair down to her neck. She has a little blue bow that holds her hair straight. She has brown eyes and she smiles at me. But it's not a happy smile. She looks like she pities me or maybe it's a look of concern. She is the only one in the room who actually looks at me. She stops right in front of the clothes rack and asks, "Do you need any help?" I do, but I can take care of myself. I can find my way out of this store. I don't know this girl anyway. I reply, "No, I'm okay." She then turns around and walks away. Within seconds, she disappears into the mall.

I didn't even have a chance to ask her what her name was. Who was she? Why does she want to help me? Does she know me? What am I doing in that store? Why can't I get up the nerve to get out from underneath the clothes rack? Why do I keep having this dream? What does it mean?

1

STAND AND DELIVER

Summer 1999 – Age 25

My teammates knew something was wrong when instead of diving for a ball down the right field line, I played it off the bounce. That wasn't like me at all. My buddy Steve, who'd nicknamed me "Pigpen" because of the way I hustled and got covered with dirt every time we stepped on the softball field, noticed it. "You look a step slow tonight," he remarked.

I knew it too. Though I'd gone four-for-four that night with a home run and made the defensive play to end the game, I was winded and weary. I struggled for breath and felt I was dragging a 40-pound weight with me when I ran the bases. I could have called it quits, claimed I was recovering from a cold and wasn't up to speed. Or I could have told the truth: Guys, I have to tell you that I have cystic fibrosis, and for the first time in a very long time, I'm afraid it's beating me. I'm terrified.

But I didn't do that either.

Though there's no love lost between me and doctors and hospitals, I knew enough to know that I needed to see a doctor. My recent decline wasn't normal – or was it? The staff at Dr. Cohen and Dr. Smith's* office ran the usual spirometry tests to see how effectively my lungs were functioning. Because cystic fibrosis causes the body to produce a thick mucus that clogs the lungs, checking lung function in a CFer (what we people with CF call ourselves) is the best way to determine his or her health.

I'm proud that I always show superb lung capacity, but this time, Dr. Smith said, "Your numbers have gone down." In fact, they'd dropped by 30 percent, which was frightening.

"What do you think it is?" I asked. I wasn't sure I wanted to know.

"Well, it could be pseudomonas."

Oh my God. That's the last word a CFer wants to hear. To a CFer, pseudomonas is the equivalent of Kryptonite to Superman. It's a potentially fatal bacteria that has been the cause of death for many CFers. Once it enters your lungs, it gradually destroys lung function and you die. I knew this because I'd been reading about cystic fibrosis while researching this book. I knew exactly what I was up against – or I would, once the results of Dr. Smith's tests came back. That could take four or five days, he said. In the interim, he prescribed some new medicines and told me to

---

*Many of the names in this book have been changed in order to protect those individuals' privacy.

do my chest therapy twice a day instead of daily.

As soon as I got to the parking lot, I sat in my car and called my mom. "My numbers are down. The doctor said it could be pseudomonas," I told her. She knew what pseudomonas was. I tried to take a deep breath, but I couldn't hold back my tears.

"Andy, it's O.K. It's not pseudomonas," my mom said.

"What if it is?" I cried. "I don't want to die, Mom. It's beating me."

"It's not," she insisted. She refused to consider otherwise, which scared me, too. She didn't know any more than I did.

After we hung up, I kept crying. I wondered where I might have picked up pseudomonas. There was no way to tell. At the CF event I volunteered for? The doctor's office? I began to drive, but I didn't know where I was going and I didn't care. Then I caught three words in a song on the radio: stand and deliver. I realized that was what I had to do. I wasn't going to let CF get the best of me.

On my way to the clinic to get my culture for pseudomonas done, I passed the hospital where I was born 25 years ago. When I was born, the doctors didn't give me much of a chance of surviving and yet here I was. I'd spent my life listening to people's dire statements and then proving them wrong. This just had to be another one of those times.

After the clinic, I headed to the gym to work out. I told myself I'd exercise every day until I got the results.

I knew exercise would help keep me sane. Unfortunately, playing softball, my favorite sport, was out. I'd been playing for the past six seasons and had never missed a game. But Dr. Smith had warned me that exposure to Atlanta's current intense humidity had to be limited now whether or not I had pseudomonas. I couldn't risk hurting myself even more. I wondered if I'd be able to play anymore this season...or ever again.

Now all I had was the gym. I shot some baskets and then told myself that if I made a full-court shot, that was a sign that I'd be fine no matter what. I heaved the ball about 90 feet and it swished neatly through the net. Just coincidence, right? Maybe. I needed something to believe in, though. I had never been so scared.

The next morning, I awoke with a throbbing throat. I called in sick at work and spent the morning in bed. Ross, my roommate, looked in to check on me. I told him what was going on and how scared I was. I expected him to pity me or just walk away from my situation...but he didn't. He told me that I was an inspiration to him and I couldn't just lie there. It was as if I was his Santa Claus. Someone to believe in. Someone that had to exist to make his life complete. I couldn't seem to get up, though.

As I turned over my troubles in my head, I realized this felt familiar. I was alone. I was feeling sorry for myself. I was lying in bed while the rest of the world was in action. What was going on? Then it hit me. I could have been back in my college fraternity room again at one of the lowest points of my life. I didn't want to go back there ever. I had to get up and get into action. I took a shower and headed in to work. Was it a coincidence that the song playing on the radio in my car was "Stand and Deliver"?

I had a tough letter to write. I had to e-mail my three softball team captains and let them know I'd be sidelined for several weeks. I could have lied about the reason but I decided to tell them I had cystic fibrosis. None of them had known.

I was overwhelmed by their support. Steve wrote back, "I'll be praying for you, buddy. When you are back in three weeks, and you will be back, I expect you to take your normal spot in the order." That brought me to tears. So did Ross's vow that if I couldn't drink for a few weeks, neither would he. And coming from a good friend like Ross, that was a big deal.

Then all there was to do was wait. And wait. Every time the phone rang, I jumped. I couldn't sleep. I couldn't concentrate. Monday and Tuesday went by slowly. On Wednesday, I got an e-mail titled "pseudomonas." My heart skipped a beat as I opened it, but it was someone I met over a chat-line, informing me that pseudomonas had been diagnosed in her son and he had to spend two weeks in the hospital. I wrote back and asked what symptoms he'd had – I wanted to know for myself, honestly. None, she responded; it was discovered during a routine office visit. That really scared me. My aunt, Susie, had reassured me that I couldn't have pseudomonas because I looked so healthy and was in such good shape. What if I had to be hospitalized? Atlanta didn't have a CF clinic. Where would I go? Why should a 25 year old have to worry about these things?

Later that day, my father entered my office. He does that a lot because I work in the business he started. This time, he took a deep breath. Oh God, I thought, he's got the results. "O.K.," he said, "tell me if I'm reading this Spanish correctly." False alarm. He was reviewing something I'd translated for him for his Spanish-speaking warehouse employees.

Wednesday night I slept a total of about 90 minutes. I woke up constantly from nightmares. I dreamed that the doctors told me I could never play sports again. They said they were sending me to a hospital far away. They told me I was going to die. I was sweating and coughing, coughing and sweating like I did during those horrible days in college.

I was exhausted by Thursday morning. And I was frustrated. Still no results. My dad and I went to lunch. He asked why I wasn't as brave as I used to be. It wasn't that I wasn't brave, I said. It's just that I didn't know what to be brave about. I still didn't know what was wrong with me. What was my enemy: pseudomonas or some other less dangerous infection? I needed to know.

I came home Thursday around 2:30. I was wiped out. I thought about the changes I'd make in my life if everything turned out to be fine. I wouldn't obsess so much over my softball statistics and winning. I'd just enjoy the game and the camaraderie. I wouldn't take my friends or family for granted. Was it too late to do those things? I hoped not, I thought as I finally fell into a fitful sleep.

I was awakened by a ringing phone. It was Dr. Cohen – finally. I thought that when his call came, I'd be terrified, but I wasn't. I just wanted to know. He told me, and finally I knew what I was facing.

2

WHAT I'M DEALING WITH

Summer 1999 – Age 25

I've accepted the fact CF doesn't just go away no matter how well I take care of myself or how much I despise it. I will wrestle with it my entire life, just as I've done for the past 25 years. I wish it would lay low and allow me to do all the stuff I want to do, but it doesn't.

I was having trouble breathing during softball games and wasn't playing my best. I kept coughing. I felt lousy despite working out and doing my therapy. I began to get scared – scared enough to see Dr. Smith, who told me he'd find out if I had pseudomonas, a serious infection. Dr. Cohen was my primary physician in Atlanta and I knew he would call with the results. Waiting to hear the test results made the week drag and made me dwell on all sorts of negative things: What if I had to go to the hospital? Would my friends visit? I'd hate for them to see me like that, but I'd feel even worse if they stayed away. My twenty-sixth birth-day was just a month away. How would it feel to spend it in the hospital?

Dr. Cohen, who is always straightforward with me, was finally on the phone. He was the kind of guy who wasn't simply your doctor. He was like family in many ways. Every time I came in for a visit, he'd talk about women he wanted to set me up with. He never actual-ly set me up, but it was a nice break from our lengthy CF discussions. I took a deep breath, which seemed to last for minutes. But if you were going to hear bad news, Dr. Cohen was the one to hear it from. He is as positive of a doctor as you'll ever meet. In past visits, the man had told me I was in better shape than him. Finally Dr. Cohen spoke: "You're going to be O.K. You have some bacteria growing, none of which is life-threatening. You've also got staph. That's why it's tough to breathe."

I was overjoyed, as were my folks, but I knew I had another fight ahead of me. Dr. Smith increased my inhaler use to twice a day, which helped but made my throat ache. I couldn't stop coughing and I had trouble breathing. I didn't mind missing a few days of work. What really bothered me was taking several weeks off from softball season.

I reluctantly told my teammates. They couldn't have been more supportive. Many called every day to see how I was doing. One of the teams sent a "get well" card that everyone signed. I read it before I worked out in the afternoon and again before I went to sleep. I eased back into working out five days a week. Some days I was exhausted and coughed up chunks of phlegm. People at the gym stared at me, but after more than a quarter-century on this planet, I was used to it. I wasn't going to let it stop me.

Still, I was scared to go back on that softball field. That's where I had first felt sick and that was my last memory of softball. Tuesday night rolled around and I had to decide if I was going to miss my sixth straight week of softball or if I was going to suck it up and get back out there. I decided I would play it safe and rest. My confidence was shaky. Then the e-mail popped up. I had written a bunch of e-mail friends and told them that I might play that night. A little girl who had CF and who had in the past told me that I was her hero said, "Hit a homer for me." Pigpen was back!

I had given CF more credit than it probably deserved. I laced up my cleats, grabbed my bat and glove, and drove to the field. When I arrived, my teammates welcomed me back with hugs, slaps on the back, and hearty handshakes. I wanted to cry because it felt so good to be part of the team again and it felt so good to be back doing what I love.

When it was my turn at bat, my friend Ira, the third-base coach, told me that as soon as I hit the ball, he'd send me home. I laughed. I didn't care so much about hitting a homer. I was happy just to be playing again. I didn't mourn losing a little bit of my competitive edge because, in exchange, I'd gained some perspective. I had, however, promised a little girl that I would hit a home run that night...

My teammates were chanting "An-dy! An-dy! An-dy!" as I stepped up to the plate. I adjusted my grip on the bat. The ball sailed toward me. I whacked it as hard as I could. I hustled to first and then second. Where was the ball? I looked at Ira, and he yelled at me to run home, just like he said he would. I touched the plate and was mobbed by teammates celebrating my home run.

O.K., so the stuff I said about losing some of my competitive edge was a lie. I can't deny that I want to win and I push myself to be the best I can. I'm not happy any other way. But I can't say that it's a bad thing. If I didn't have that drive, I might have given up against CF a long time ago. Instead, I was alive at 25. Something no one would have guessed 25 years earlier.

3

PARENTAL GUIDANCE

Fall 1973 – Birth

Not long after I was born on September 4, 1973, the doctors discovered that I had a blocked intestine, a symptom of cystic fibrosis. The odds I'd have this serious genetic disease were one in four because my parents were both carriers. I was that one.

We didn't talk about cystic fibrosis when I was little. I knew it wasn't something everyone had, and I knew it wasn't really something anyone wanted. Other than having my parents administer therapy – every day they had to pound on my chest to release the thick mucus from my lungs – I didn't think too much about it. Of course, back then, I didn't know much and I didn't know what to ask.

When I was in grade school, my mother made what I consider to be one of the most important decisions about my life. We were at the hospital for my monthly checkup with Dr. Compton*, who looked perpetually concerned about my health. My mom called him a "pessimistic" doctor. But then again, there weren't too many doctors, who were optimistic, about the outlook for a cystic fibrosis child. He and my mom chatted, and then Dr. Compton suggested she send me to cystic fibrosis camp.

That's where, I learned, kids with this life-threatening disorder could get together and talk about CF. The reality of CF is that some of these kids wouldn't survive five years. Others might not even make it a year. And others, well, they might live for decades. The risk in attending a CF camp was the possibility of catching a serious bacterial illness such as pseudomonas. Everyone is tested before they enroll, but that's no guarantee against infection. If one camper was affected, pseudomonas could easily spread to everyone, with possibly fatal consequences.

Dr. Compton knew this, but he told my mom that the benefits outweighed the risks. He recommended I attend the camp to meet other kids who knew how it felt to receive therapy each day and learn how they handled the challenges of CF.

It sounded good to me. I just wanted to go to camp and play with my fellow campers, whether they had CF or not. I didn't know of any of the dangers that came along with attending these camps. I figured my mom would say yes. After all, she and my dad were big contributors to CF charities. My mom headed the Santa

Claus House, an annual fundraiser for the CF Foundation, and my dad was on the board of CF Foundation camps in Georgia, including the one that Dr. Compton mentioned.

My mom considered Dr. Compton's recommendation. She looked at me, but I don't think she was asking me to decide. Then she walked with him to a corner in the room and, as she would tell me later, she softly said, "I'd prefer that he didn't go. I don't want Andy to become friends with kids he'll see pass away. I don't want him to think he's different from everyone else just because he has CF. I want him to have a normal life. He deserves that opportunity."

That might seem ironic in light of my parents' support of CF groups, but my mom felt there were some CF children who needed CF camp and others who didn't. I fell in the latter category.

It was unusual. Dr. Compton had told my mom what I couldn't eat and what I couldn't do athletically. So many times, Dr. Compton had told my mother and me about the things I could not do. On this day, she was telling him that I could accomplish a lot. She wouldn't allow CF to define and/or limit me. She wanted me to be a kid like every other kid.

And yet, when I entered grade school, I became known for being small, weak and often ill. My parents didn't trust me to take my medication. It wasn't because I was a bad kid, but it was the fact that I was a kid. So every day during lunch, I went to the principal's office to get my medication. My friends asked me why I went to the principal's office, but I just told them that my mom left my lunch there. Without those pills, I couldn't eat lunch, so technically I wasn't lying.

It was important that my teachers know I had CF in case of a medical emergency. Even if my classmates didn't know I had cystic fibrosis, they quickly figured out that I was such a poor athlete that no one wanted me on their team. I finished last when we had to run laps in gym class. Sometimes it took me so long that the gym teacher would tell me not to finish because everyone else was ready to move on to another activity. My parents didn't seem too concerned about this. When I was sick (and even when I wasn't), my mom would write a note to the gym teacher asking that I be excused because of cystic fibrosis. At the time, the notes were a relief. I didn't have to embarrass myself that day. But looking back, I wish she had never written them. The excuses moved from my mom's letters to constants in my mind.

Over the years, my classmates learned that I had CF. I doubt any of them knew much about it, but when you're a kid, any sign of difference is perceived as bad, and you become a target. Some kids taunted me by saying I'd be dead before I ever got to high school. One girl, Julie, used to grab my frail arm and say, "You're so skinny!" I'd come home many days and cry. My mom, though, told me that everything was fine. I didn't know who or what to believe. My mom had always been there for me, but she had always been so adamant about me taking pills. She would ask me every day after school if I took them. It made me realize that if I didn't, something negative would happen to me. So I began to believe my friends.

I missed a lot of school. Kids get the sniffles and colds a lot, and that's perfectly normal, but it can be more serious for someone who has cystic fibrosis, so my mom was especially vigilant. I hated it. Sometimes I missed weeks of school. Being home was worse than being picked on in school. I used to sit inside with Howard, my dog, and watch enviously as the other kids played ball outside, sometimes even in my yard. No one ever asked me to play. When my mom did let me go outside, it was always with a stern warning to be careful and not overexert myself. My mom wanted me to have a life, but she had a lot of fears. What if something happened to me? What if she couldn't be there? Maybe she was contradicting her decision to forbid me to attend CF camp. Bet she was a mom and that gave her the right to worry.

I spent my afternoons parked in front of the TV watching cartoons and sitcoms. I must've watched about six hours of TV a day. I couldn't do anything else, and the shows, with their laugh tracks and easily resolved problems, were my way of escaping reality. Unlike my dad, TV never yelled at me or expected anything from me.

Every night when my father came home, he'd ask

what I did that day. He wasn't pleased to learn that I'd spent another afternoon glued to the screen.

"You need to go outside," he said. "You need to play with your friends."

As if I had any friends. No one wanted to play with me. I didn't want to tell that to my dad, though, because I thought he'd be even more disappointed in me. I often had the sense that my dad expected more from me than I knew how to give. I thought of the dads I'd seen on TV, happily playing catch with their sons and dispensing wise advice, fixing everything that was wrong. I wasn't anything like those freckle-faced kids. I feared my dad regretted having such a sickly, skinny kid and didn't love me. And perhaps I was disappointed too, disappointed that my dad, who seemed to be able to handle any situation and fix any problem, couldn't fix me. I was his child, wasn't I? Wasn't there anything he could do? Didn't he see how unhappy I was?

The tension in my family about CF came to a head when I was about 7 years old. I had to write a report on Christopher Columbus. I hated book reports; they always got in the way of "The Brady Bunch." I wanted an easy way out, so I asked my father who Christopher Columbus was. He looked disappointed and said he wasn't going to help me. "That's why I bought the encyclopedias in the den," he said. "You know how to use them."

I trudged into the den and pulled the "C" volume off the shelf. I opened the book and began turning pages. Before I discovered Columbus, though, I saw the entry for "cystic fibrosis." I shouldn't have been surprised to find it there – hey, it *was* an encyclopedia – but I was. My parents had always censored what I read and watched in order to limit what I knew about CF. Doctors gave us videotapes about CF, but my mom never let me watch them. She said I didn't need to see them though the doctors had made it clear they were for me, too. I was a little afraid to ask why. I didn't want to upset my mother.

So that night I began to read about cystic fibrosis. There wasn't a lot of information. I learned that CF affects the lungs and pancreas and makes mucus thicken. I skipped the long, boring medical words. Then my eye caught a sentence. After I read it, I wished I'd skipped that too. It said: "Cystic fibrosis patients normally die before the age of 25." So this is what my parents were hiding from me. The kids at school were right. I was going to die. I began to cry.

I went back to the living room and tearfully asked my parents, "Am I going to die?"

"Where did you hear that?" my mom asked. She probably suspected kids at school had been taunting me, and she could tell me to ignore them. This time, though, my information came from the encyclopedia they'd bought and kept in the house.

I told my parents I hated them. I hated cystic fibrosis. I told them I wished I was dead. I really didn't; I just threw that in because death was on my mind. My mother began bawling and ran upstairs. I don't think she'd ever seen me disagree with her so viciously. My father got angry and told me to apologize to my mother. Apologize for what? The fact that I had already lived more than a quarter of my life? The fact that I was only a second-grader and I knew I was going to die?

I began to sob and ran upstairs to my room. I sat in the dark and cried. I kept thinking about the article, the facts right there in black and white. My parents had lied to me, putting on a happy face and allowing me to think I could lead a normal life with cystic fibrosis. That was obviously not true.

Eventually, my sobs quieted and I overheard my parents discussing the situation. I couldn't hear their words, but my father's tone was one of anger and disgust, and my mother sounded very defensive.

That night might have been the first time I had the dream about the mysterious girl in the mall who wanted to know if I needed help. Who was she and why did she care? She looked so worried. I was sitting under a clothes rack and she asked me if I needed her help. Why would I need help? I don't need help. Then she vanished.

Early the next morning I awoke to a familiar voice.

"Get dressed," my father said. "We're going."

"No, I'm tired," I said from my bed, barely opening my eyes. "Leave me alone."

"Andy, get your butt out of bed," he said in a voice that meant business. "We're leaving."

I thought he might be throwing me out of the house for upsetting my mom. Where would I live?

"Where are we going?" I asked nervously. It was Saturday morning and I was eager for the lineup of my favorite cartoons. My morning was spoken for – if he let me stay.

"Baseball tryouts," my dad said. "It's time you went outside and learned to play sports. You'll thank me one day."

Who was he kidding? The only thing I knew about sports were the rules. I certainly couldn't play. I had no strength or stamina. Why didn't my father just accept that as much as he wanted me to be like other sons, I wasn't?

"I don't want to go," I said, suddenly wide-awake. "I can't play sports! Mom!"

My dad was unmoved. "Let's go," he said, pulling back the covers and tugging me out of bed.

I thought my mom would try to talk my dad out of this crazy scheme because she feared I'd get sick or be hurt. But she didn't say anything. Maybe she really was mad at me. Did she want me to die?

Our first stop was the mall, where my dad bought me a baseball glove. Then we drove to the field. It was dazzling green, or at least it looked that way through my puffy bloodshot eyes. There were lots of other boys with their parents. The coach told us to form lines so he could watch us run, catch, throw, and hit. It sounded like gym class to me, and that didn't sound good.

I was the slowest, most awkward kid on the field. When a ball came toward me, I ducked. I wasn't sure which hand to wear my glove on. The coaches yelled at me, and the other kids laughed. I swung wildly at balls, but didn't hit a thing. As the humiliations mounted, I kept glancing at my dad for a sign that he'd seen enough and we could go home. He didn't. He told me to stay out there. Whenever I swung the bat, he'd offer the same advice: "Keep your eye on the ball." I wasn't sure what that meant.

After 90 minutes that seemed like an eternity, try-outs were over. I walked with my head down, looking at the grass that had looked so beautiful when I first walked out. Now it wasn't even noticeable. I finally made it to the car and didn't say a word on the way home. What was there to say – that I let my dad down once again? That he'd finally seen proof that I was as uncoordinated a son as any man could have? I knew I couldn't be good enough for him. I wished he wasn't my dad. Why did I feel so frustrated? Why did I care?

Slowly it came to me that, yes, I did care. It mattered to me that I couldn't do something well, and I wanted to change that. It was different from gym class. That was only about what my teachers and classmates thought. This was about my dad, someone I looked up to for approval, someone I loved...despite occasional spells of thinking the contrary. When I was on the base-ball field that morning, my mom couldn't excuse me with a note. My father could have taken me home, but he watched me and wouldn't let me leave. Instead of feeling angry at him, I felt disappointed and disgusted with myself and furious at the kids who'd ridiculed me. I wanted to change the way things were. I just wasn't sure how.

That night for the first time, I joined my dad in the den as he watched the Braves game on TV. There were players doing the same maneuvers on the field that I'd tried that day. They made it look so graceful and easy the way they snagged a soaring ball in their glove or sent a ball sailing deep into the outfield. I saw my dad smile when he watched them. I wanted my father to smile like that when he saw me on the field.

That night I couldn't sleep. After my parents went to bed, I grabbed my new mitt and a tennis ball and snuck into the basement. It was a spooky place, a dark and unfinished room with shadowy corners that hid crickets, spider webs and who knew what else? I made Howard come with me just in case Freddy Krueger showed up.

I wanted to show the guys on the field that I could play just as well as they did. In fact, even better. I wanted to earn their respect and my father's. I had a ways to go. I threw the ball against the basement wall and tried to catch it the way the Major League players did. I missed. I dove, leaped, and ran for the ball. I missed again and again. I felt more and more frustrated, envisioning everyone laughing at me. I threw the ball about 200 times before Howard and I snuck up to bed.

The next day, I did the same thing. I had scraped-up knees and bruised shins, and sometimes I cut my elbows diving for balls. But I wouldn't let myself leave until I caught the ball and threw the ball a little better each time.

I'd like to say that all that determination paid off. Truthfully, though, I was still the worst player on the team. Granted, I didn't duck when a ball sailed in my direction, but I usually couldn't catch it either. When I was up at bat, I didn't hold the bat and wait for the ball to hit it. I actually swung. Not that I got any hits, but I was getting the hang of the game. I was still the last one picked for anything, but I knew I was improving. I sure couldn't have gotten much worse.

Sometimes I'd play catch with my father. He would hit one towering fly ball after another until I caught one. He'd say, "You'll never get this one!" That would make me try even harder. We also watched Braves games together and cheered on our team. That was the most fun I ever had with my dad. It was my way of showing him that I wanted to please him. Baseball became my way of telling my dad he could be proud of me. I knew I was no All-Star my first couple of Little League seasons. I vowed that the third one would be different.

4

PROVING

Summer 1982 - Age 9

The next summer when my Little League team, the Zephyrs, ran onto the field for opening day, I prayed I'd have a better season than I did with the Yankees and Knights. That wouldn't have taken much. I hadn't seen third base at all the two seasons before. Heck, second could have been a mirage for all I knew. So it was ironic that the coach positioned me at second base.

I glanced into the stands and spotted my parents among the crowd of chatting moms and dads. I didn't want to embarrass them. I wanted my dad to say proudly, "See the second baseman? That's my son, Andy." I hoped to show him how much I'd improved and how far I'd come as an athlete.

The first batter positioned himself by the tee, which the coaches always used for the first game of the season. He took a few practice swings as I grew increasingly edgy. Finally, he swung the bat, which made a loud "Crack!" when it connected solidly with the ball. I noticed with a mix of excitement and fear that that very same ball was headed straight for me.

I leaped as high as my 10-year-old body could lift me and raised my gloved hand to meet the ball. When my feet hit the ground, I noticed the crowd was silent. The batter had stopped running toward first base. "Great," I thought. "I'm so bad that the runner actually had to stop and laugh."

I glanced into my glove, which to this point had been used only as a wig for the pumpkin lady my mom and I made each Halloween. Nestled inside was a large spherical object with red stitching running around it, a baseball. And it was in my possession. I'd finally caught a ball. All those rigorous practices, scraped knees, bruised elbows, and carpet burns had finally paid off.

But the best memory of the day came a second later. I looked into the stands and saw one man stand up and applaud like his kid had hit a home run with the bases loaded in the bottom of the ninth with the score tied. He hollered "All right, Andy!" so loudly that I had no trouble hearing him on the field. My dad was so proud of me that he proclaimed to everyone that I was his son.

I was building the confidence that cystic fibrosis had been tearing down. And I was changing my relationship with my dad. I realized that the reason he'd sent me to Little League tryouts two years before was not to humiliate me. Instead, he wanted to show me that if I worked hard, I could play well, just like anyone else. He didn't want me to use CF as an excuse for not trying or excelling.

My dad also introduced me to tennis. Again, I learned that hard work pays off. I began to practice every day, hitting the ball with my father, my mother, Aunt Susie and Uncle Bobby. My mom enrolled me at the Atlanta Jewish Community Center's tennis camp. I was disappointed to find that when we were grouped by skill, I was in the lowest level and all my friends were in the highest level. Playing with the kids in my group, I got really tired of going into the woods every five minutes to retrieve tennis balls. I hadn't seen that many balls sail over a fence since I watched highlights of Hank Aaron's career. But I kept practicing and eventually was moved up to the highest level with my friends. Just before camp ended our instructor, Fran, announced that we'd play a round-robin tournament. The champion at each level would receive a trophy. As soon as she said the word "trophy," I knew I really wanted it.

That night I was tossing a tennis ball against the living room wall repeatedly to prepare for the upcoming baseball season. (I'd had to move my practice field from the basement after finding a baby snake down there.) My mom had told me a zillion times not to play ball in the living room – isn't that a standard Momism? – but of course I didn't listen. I had a pretty accurate arm and hadn't broken any of her good china or knickknacks. Yet.

That day, I made a toss about three inches to the right of the wall. The ball sailed into a vase, knocking it onto the tile floor. It shattered into a thousand pieces. I couldn't believe it. What was I going to tell my mom?

There was nothing to tell her because as soon as she saw that her favorite vase was missing, she knew what happened. She spanked me and sent me to bed without television. I cried for hours. I wanted to make her feel guilty, but she knew that trick. The next morning, she told me how disappointed she was.

"Fine," I sulked. "Punish me more. I won't play in the tennis tournament. Are you happy now?"

She looked at me and said something I'll never forget. "You'd better play," she said, "because you are going to win and put the trophy where the vase used to be." Then she grinned and gave me a hug.

The day of the tournament, I felt infused with motivation. I was going to return home with a trophy and put a smile on my mom's face. My first opponent was Graham, who I was pretty confident I could beat. And I did, four games to one. That wasn't too bad.

But then I had to face Adam, last year's tournament winner and an undefeated player at camp. I'd lost to him five times already and had only just racked up my first win, against Graham. I was nervous. Something peculiar happened in that first game, though: I won. I'm still not sure how. But all the butterflies left my stomach and confidence flowed into my head. I remembered that my mother wanted me to

win the trophy, and I wanted to win it for her. I was-
n't leaving without it. We finished our set. Adam won
three games. I won five.

My last competitor was my best friend, Josh, who
I'd never beaten. He hadn't seen my match against
Adam and asked how I did. When I told him I'd beat-
en Adam, his eyes widened. "Are you kidding?" he
said. I told him I'd played the best I ever played. That,
of course, motivated Josh to want to beat me. I was the
last of the undefeated players. We ended up splitting
our match with three games each. I'd never beaten Josh
before, so that was a victory, too.

Tired and sweaty, we gathered around Fran as
Adam's dad, one of the camp's volunteers, punched our
results into his calculator. The trophy would go to whoever won the highest percentage of games. The drizzle
that was falling while I was playing Adam had become
a light shower. Judging from the dark clouds overhead,
it was getting ready to pour. Fran went into her office
for the trophy. I was so nervous that my hands were
shaking and my stomach ached. The rain began to fall
faster. Finally, Adam's dad was finished.

"Adam won a total of 13 of 21 games," he said.
"And Andy won 12 of 19."

Darn. I lost by a game. That's not fair; I beat him.
My mom gave me a hug, but I pushed her away. "Why
are you hugging me?" I said. "I lost."

"No, you didn't," she said.

Adam's father continued: "That means Andy won

63 percent of his games. Adam won 62 percent. Congratulations, Andy."

Oh my gosh! I won. Fran handed me the most beautiful trophy I'd ever seen. Sure, it was plastic and the inscription was a little blurry, but it was mine. I earned it. It was pouring now, and my mom and I ran to the car. I told my mom we could put it on the table where the vase used to stand, and she smiled.

Eventually I developed a collection of about 30 trophies. I picked up more while playing Little League (I became the starting first baseman for my teams) and tennis (I was the top singles player on every team and had a 30-match winning streak). I also played football and basketball. That's not to say I was the world's best athlete. There were a lot of kids who were better than me. But I steadily improved, and that tennis trophy I earned years ago is a reminder of that. If my parents' house were to go up in flames, I'd dash in to grab that. It's more than just a plastic memento; it's a reminder that someone who wasn't given much of a chance triumphed due to perseverance, skill, and support.

A lot of that support came from my parents. They cheered me on and urged me to do the best I could, and they never let CF be my excuse for not trying. They saw their efforts pay off. My mom no longer had to write me excuse notes for gym class. Now I was running laps around my classmates. I didn't think CF could ever defeat me. That is... until I saw Alex.

5

MY KINSHIP
WITH ALEX

Fall 1985 – Age 12

My parents usually watched TV at night before they went to bed. Well, I shouldn't say "watched" because most nights, the TV was background noise while they talked to each other or chatted on the phone. After I was finished with my homework, I'd often join them and watch the conclusion of whatever show they were watching – or, more often, weren't watching.

One night when I was about 12, I noticed something unusual before I even entered their bedroom. Standing in the doorway, I could see them both focused intently on the screen. That was odd. If what they were watching was so good, why hadn't they called me in so I could see it, too?

I held very still, trying to figure out what was going on and hoping that my parents wouldn't notice me. I spotted something strange in bed – a box of tissues nestled between my parents. At the commercial break, my mom grabbed a tissue, wiped her eyes and blew her nose. There was already a little pile of wadded-up tissues on the night table by her side of the bed. What the heck was going on?

When the show resumed, I sneaked a glance at the screen and saw something I'd never seen before: a girl using the same type of aerosol therapy that I used. She was also getting the same type of therapy my parents gave me. It was about time, I thought. Finally I'd seen someone who knew what my life was like. She looked like a really nice girl, too, someone I could be friends with, maybe. She reminded me of the girl who kept reappearing in my dream. The girl in the shopping mall. The one who kept asking if I needed any help. I wondered if this girl was her. Then I saw something that completely disrupted my thinking. Doubled over in pain, this cute girl began to cough up blood, gasp, and cry in pain.

At that minute, my mother glanced over at the door. She looked almost guilty. "Go to your room and go to bed!" she yelled. "You don't need to be watching this. This is an adult movie!"

That was exactly what I needed to hear. Anything that I shouldn't be watching was something that I wanted to see, especially if it involved someone with CF.

"But I want to watch it," I pleaded.

"Go to bed!" she hollered. It was clear that arguing wasn't an option.

I had another plan, though. I obediently went into my room and shut the door. I switched on the television in my bedroom and turned down the volume so my parents wouldn't hear the sound. There was the girl, this time looking very frail, lying in bed, her parents at her side. They were sobbing. What the heck was going on?

Before I could catch up with the story, my mother came storming in. She was still crying, and her mascara made black smears down her face. She clicked off the TV and ordered me to bed.

The next morning, everything was "normal." We didn't talk about the show or what happened to the girl or why my parents were crying. But I wasn't stupid. I began to worry that like the girl in the movie, I too would cough up blood and become bed-ridden. No one could live like that, so I knew I would die. Would it be terrible like that? What ever happened to her? Would the same thing happen to me? These questions plagued me for years. I'd be lying if I didn't admit that sometimes they still haunt me.

It took me more than 13 years to find out who the girl was and what happened to her. I'd started writing this book and was looking on the Internet for information about CF. I found a Website that mentioned Frank Deford, a *Sports Illustrated* writer. His name was familiar to me because I remembered my mom telling me that he was involved in the Cystic Fibrosis Foundation and had lost a daughter who had CF. I double-clicked on his name and read his biography. It mentioned a book he'd written *Alex: The Life of a Child*, which had been made into a movie. Aha.

Looking back, I think my mom did the right thing in not letting me watch the movie. My parents tried to shelter me as much as possible from the negative stuff about CF so that I could enjoy my childhood without fearing for my life and obsessing about my health. I remember how my mom would tell me to just ignore the kids in elementary school who taunted me about dying from CF. I remembered how she refused to enroll me in CF camp because she didn't want me to be around kids who were sicker than I was and who might get me focused on illness and dying.

But I think I would have been better off if I'd known a little more about CF. As a kid, I didn't know anyone else who had cystic fibrosis. Imagine being African-American and growing up without seeing another black person. Or imagine speaking French and for years never encountering another French speaker. You'd start to think you were not "normal" without realizing there was a universe where you fit right in. You'd assume there must be other people like you. You'd long to meet them just to "compare notes," to reinforce the idea that you're part of a group, and to know that the things that you feel, other people feel them too. That was absent from my childhood and teen years. It made those times, which are tough for every kid, even more alienating for me.

There was no one I could talk to about cystic fibrosis. I mean, I could have talked to my parents or my doctors, but that was different. First, neither of them knew what it was like to have CF. Second, my parents were afraid to tell me anything about CF and I was afraid the doctors would tell me too much. Not that that's a bad thing. My parents tried to be optimistic, and the doctors, I think, were pessimistic, especially when they talked about the long term.

Though I'd never met Frank Deford or read the book he'd written about his daughter, Alex, I had a hunch that he would understand a lot of my feelings. I sent him a note telling him about my book's purpose and how much I appreciated his leadership efforts with CF. I asked him if he'd write a foreword. Hey, why not?

I didn't expect a response. After all, the guy is a famous sportswriter who probably gets a lot of mail and keeps a busy schedule. So I was very surprised several weeks later to find a note from him in the mail. He wrote that he was touched by my story and would be pleased to write a few words for the beginning of my book. So that explains how his foreword appears in this book.

If he was going to do that for me, the least I could do was read his book. I bought it and kept it unopened for several weeks. I knew it had a sad ending: a beloved daughter dies of CF. I finally cracked the cover on an insanely early flight to Cincinnati for one of my routine doctor's appointments. I was exhausted from a late night softball game the night before. Once I started reading, however, I couldn't put Alex's story down. So much in her life mirrored mine.

Like me, she'd thought about death, but was afraid to talk about it with her parents. Like me, she was disappointed and depressed because she couldn't keep up with her friends in gym class. She, too, loved her closest friends because they didn't treat her any differently because of CF. And both of us knew what it was like to have cystic fibrosis.

Alex wasn't expected to live longer than a couple of years, but she proved the doctors wrong. I admired her so much for that, for fighting for her life and never giving up. She lived eight years, and her death, though tragic, had a dramatic impact on the country's awareness of CF. Before Alex's story was shared with the nation, the CF Foundation was raising about $15 million a year. Following the release of the book and movie about Alex's life, that amount leapt to $130 million for research. So it's due to Alex, really, and the Defords that I'm as healthy as I am today. I owe her big time.

One of my goals is to finish what Alex started. I want to change the perception that people have about CF patients. Yes, it's a deadly disease, but the breakthroughs that occur nearly every day put CF closer than ever to a cure. I also want people to know that individuals with CF should not be treated differently. As Frank Deford put it so well: "If you start off saying a child is special because she suffers from a handicap, that is a disservice, because you are robbing her of what she might become on her own." He's right.

I never thought I'd consider an 8-year-old girl a hero. After all, what can a child accomplish? In Alex's case, a lot more than most adults. Thanks, kid.

6

MY HIGH SCHOOL TENNIS DAYS

Spring 1988 – Age 14

Anyone who went to my high school, Dunwoody High, knew that it had an amazing tennis team. The year before I started school there, the team had won the state championship and had won three of the last five titles. Tennis had been my sport since I earned that trophy at tennis camp. I'd always been the best player on my team. I knew I wanted to play varsity tennis at Dunwoody though I was "just" a freshman.

Tryouts in the spring couldn't come soon enough. They worked like this: Each player would play one elimination match. The winner would qualify for the varsity team. I signed up on the spot. The sheet posted a week later on the door of the tennis team coach, Ms. Baker*, said I'd face Jason. We'd played the top two singles positions on the same junior-level team, but we'd never played each other. I knew he was a

strong player and he wouldn't be easy to beat. I began
dreaming about the match. Sometimes I'd win.
Sometimes I'd lose. No matter what the outcome, I'd
still wake up drenched with sweat from serving and
slamming in my sleep.

The day finally arrived. My classes seemed to drag.
I couldn't pay attention because all I could think about
was the afternoon match. Maybe Jason wouldn't show.
Maybe he'd chicken out. But he didn't. When my mom
drove me to tryouts, there he was with a racket in one
hand and a water bottle in the other. My mom wished
me good luck and said she'd be watching. I was the
only guy there whose mom had driven him. That's
because most of the other guys were older and could
drive. I didn't even have a learner's permit.

Ms. Baker called our names, and we walked onto
the court. The tension was thick. I was already sweating. I visualized myself playing varsity tennis for the
defending state championship team, and I gave that
match everything I had. My game plan was to be
aggressive early on and win points at the net. I hustled
and dove. Early on, the games were tight, but as the
match wore on, I began to dominate. I defeated Jason
eight games to one. It took a minute to sink in.

I was the only ninth-grade guy to make the team.
Not just any team, but the defending state champions.
I was playing a varsity sport. I was going to have a varsity letter for my varsity jacket though I couldn't even
drive yet. I was going to make a name for myself on the

squad and be there to collect the trophy when we won yet another state title.

When I got home, I rode my yellow Huffy bike one mile to Aunt Susie and Uncle Bobby's house. They knew better than anyone what a victory on the tennis court meant to me. Before I got there, though, I saw the mailman. I had to share this amazing news, so I yelled to him, "I made the team!" I'm sure he wondered what I'd had for an afternoon snack.

Aunt Susie was as proud and excited as I'd hoped. We reminisced about how she and Uncle Bobby used to blow away my dad and me on the tennis courts and how I was always the last one picked for teams. Sharing my success with her made it seem real and made it a lot sweeter.

Unfortunately, the only euphoria I enjoyed as part of the varsity tennis team was the thrill of making the team. That first season was a nightmare. In order to play on the team that week, you had to be ranked among the top 10 players. Each week there was a challenge ladder. You could challenge any player one or two spots ahead of you. I was beaten by every player I challenged. Because I didn't beat anyone, I didn't play a single match all season. My parents came to matches, but they never saw me on the court. All I did was sit on the sidelines and watch the stronger, faster players. My only action was fetching water for my exhausted teammates. I felt like a failure having to tell my parents again each week that no, I wasn't playing this time either. It reminded me of all the times when I was the kid with CF who had to watch all his friends play sports in his own backyard.

The worst part of the season was the very end, at the awards banquet. My name wasn't even mentioned. I didn't receive a letter for my letterman's jacket, which I'd purchased. I didn't win "most improved" or "best overall" player. My parents said they were proud of me regardless. I didn't believe them. I was furious at Ms. Baker for not even acknowledging the hard work I'd put in all season. I wanted to storm out of the banquet. But my mom insisted that I shake her hand and thank her for the season. I felt bitter as I did it. She had a lot of nerve to humiliate me by inviting me to the banquet and then embarrassing me in front of my parents. Next season, I vowed, she'd realize how much she underestimated me.

I decided that if I was going to excel as a tennis player, I'd have to work extra hard. During the off-season, I began working with a tennis coach and practiced several hours a day during the week. On the weekends, I played in a junior tennis league. I knew I was getting better. I was more agile on the court and could better anticipate opponents' shots and moves. It paid off.

That following spring, I made the varsity team again, but this time, I began moving up the challenge ladder. The first week, I was ranked No. 7 out of 18 players. My teammate Josh and I won a doubles regulation match, and we played doubles together every week that season. We won every match we played and ultimately beat the defending state champions, Tucker High School. That year's awards banquet was quite different. I finally earned my letter for my jacket. I also received a plaque for my contribution to the team, and Ms. Baker acknowledged my skill and hard work. When I shook her hand at that banquet, I felt redeemed.

I played varsity tennis during all of my four years at Dunwoody. I was never one of the team's top players, but I still compiled 18 wins without a loss in competition. I went from not playing a single match my first season to three consecutive undefeated seasons. I'd say I showed Ms. Baker – and myself.

That first season on the team was a mixed blessing. It was a humiliating experience to be sidelined in a sport I thought I knew. But I learned something valuable, too. I found out what kind of a competitor I really was. I wasn't satisfied with being mediocre. Thus, I worked to excel. That approach served me well in sports, and I knew it would impact my approach to cystic fibrosis and life. Things weren't going to come easy for me. I'd have to work to achieve my goals. As I ended my senior year of high school, I realized I was just months away from one of my biggest goals – college.

7

INDEPENDENCE DAY – MY MACHINE ARRIVES

Fall 1989 – Age 16

Ask me what the most significant thing I ever received was and you might be surprised by my answer. It's not my baseball glove or my tennis trophy or my driver's license. Topping my list would be the bronchial therapy machine my parents got for me when I was 16. My mom says they had to fight with the insurance company to get them to pay for it, but it was worth the hassle.

For most 16 year olds, a car provides freedom, freedom to go where they want to go without being dependent on their parents. For me, the chest therapy machine was the equivalent. It changed my life so much you would've thought I'd gotten not just a car, but a Porsche.

Before I got this machine, my parents had administered my chest therapy every day from the time I was two weeks old. Each morning I would lie on a pillow and my father or mother would cup their hands and thump all over my chest. It made a popping sound, and the process loosened the mucus in my lungs. Then I'd have to cough it up. Great fun! I had to switch positions six times so they could cover my whole chest. And you thought having your folks make you clean your room was a hassle!

Therapy didn't necessarily hurt, but it certainly wasn't fun. And it wasted at least a half-hour of every day for me and my parents. I couldn't watch television, read, or talk. I felt trapped while they were doing the therapy. It was like waiting in five o'clock traffic while cars slowly moved through the line. It was so frustrating. Sometimes my mom would forget to take off her wedding ring, and boy, that would sting. I know it was hard for my parents as well. They'd been administering therapy to me before I even knew why it was being done. When I was an infant and toddler, they had to hold me down while I screamed and struggled.

I was always concerned that therapy would make it impossible for me to leave home. As I went through high school and my friends began visiting colleges and talking about where they'd like to go, this weighed on me more and more. I wanted to go to a university too, but I sure as heck didn't want to take my parents with me. Living at home and going to a school in Atlanta didn't really appeal to me because I wanted the "real" college experience of going to a new place and being on my own. I began to think that making good grades wasn't important...because what was the point? I wouldn't be able to attend college.

Then the bronchial therapy machine came along. It was connected to a vest that fit snugly around my chest. I'd turn on the machine, which sounded like a vacuum cleaner, and it would send currents into the vest that would vibrate my chest. I used six frequencies for five minutes each while making the vest tighter or looser. The great thing about the machine was that I could do my aerosol therapy – a mist-like treatment, which I inhaled like a nebulizer – at the same time, which shaved about 25 minutes from my routine. I could also watch TV, play video games, or even do homework during therapy. And unlike my parents, this therapy machine never nagged me to finish my homework or brush my teeth. The therapy machine was portable, too. It could be wheeled anywhere or hidden in a closet or under a bed. That meant I could go on vacations and trips with friends and didn't need my parents tagging along to administer therapy. It seemed to eliminate all limitations imposed by CF.

The machine was a relatively new invention when I got it. My parents were glad to share what they knew with other families who had a CF child. That's how I met Chris. He was planning to attend LaGrange College in Georgia, and his parents wanted to check out my bronchial therapy machine to see if it'd be a good thing for him to use in school. My dad didn't like me interacting with other CFers, but Chris didn't have and major bacterial infections. Thus, my father reluctantly accepted to us meeting. When he visited, I showed him the machine and told him how much I liked it. I even fitted him with the vest and let him try it. We talked for a few minutes, and as we did, I noticed something. Every time I tried to talk about sports or college or hobbies, Chris steered the conversation back to cystic fibrosis. He seemed preoccupied with it. It took me a little while to realize why.

We went downstairs, where our parents were talking. Chris's dad wanted to know how I liked the machine. "Does it make you feel better?" he asked.

"No," I joked, "I think it's killing me!"

But nobody laughed. I had no idea why. I always thought I was pretty funny.

"He's just kidding," my mom explained meekly.

As we talked more, I learned that Chris was having a much harder time with CF than I was. He'd been hospitalized a number of times due to complications stemming from CF. I noticed he was much skinnier than I was, and his voice was quite hoarse while mine was clear. He walked slowly, almost gingerly, while I couldn't sit still.

Meeting him made me realize that not every CFer was worried simply about attending college. Some were dealing with life-threatening questions, such as if they'd be hospitalized again and if so, for how long. My encounter with Chris helped me understand that I was, relatively speaking, in pretty good shape for someone with CF. And though I didn't like to dwell on it, my health could have been much worse and my options much more limited.

8

MY FRIEND
FOR LIFE

Fall 1991 – Age 18

I started college at the University of Georgia in the fall of 1991. Like most freshmen, I was excited about the independence I'd finally have and the friends I expected to make, but I was also nervous. In addition to the usual jitters about leaving behind high school friends and familiar surroundings, I had a bunch of CF-related concerns. What if my therapy machine got strange looks from the people in my dorm? What if I got sick? What if I had a problem with my medicine?

I'd hoped to sneak my therapy machine into the dorm, but it's hard to sneak in something that's three feet high and two feet wide with plastic hoses connected to it. I could see people whispering to each other, and I guessed at what they were saying: "Hey, look, that kid must be really sick to need something like that." "What do you think that thing is? Why does he have to bring it to school?" and "Do you think he's got something that's contagious?"

Some of my high school friends had seen the machine and asked what it was. I'd never told anyone in my high school – except my best friend Josh – that I had CF. I didn't want sympathy. And I didn't plan to tell anyone now. I said it was my computer. I doubt they believed me, but they didn't ask any more questions. I wondered if this experience was an omen, a hint of what my four years at UGA would be like...people giving me strange looks and laughing at me.

Before I left for college, my dad asked me what I wanted to study. I had no idea. Not a clue. He also asked if I thought about joining a fraternity. I admitted I didn't know much about them.

"It's like a club," my dad said, "but the members are called brothers. They're the guys who will be at your wedding and maybe even your son's bar mitzvah."

"I don't think Christie Brinkley will let me invite these guys to our wedding," I said with a laugh. "Besides, I've got lots of friends to hang out with."

"It's not the same," my dad said. "These guys are going to be your friends for life."

The way he looked at me when he said "friends for life" made me realize his fraternity – he was a Phi Epsilon Pi at the University of South Carolina – had meant a lot to him and still did. I figured I'd check it out.

I knew I already had a friend for life, Josh. Not only was he my college roommate, but he was also my tennis team doubles partner and the person who knew more about me than anyone. We agreed that if either of us decided to join a fraternity, we'd both join the same one. Josh and I have been friends since we were five. My first memory is of a kid my size with red hair and an attitude. We were going to be attending the same private school, Mount Vernon Presbyterian School, and our mothers had been put in touch with each other so they could carpool. While they got acquainted in Josh's mom's kitchen, we watched TV for 15 minutes and then got in a huge fight. Hair was pulled and punches were thrown. I cried all the way home. We've been friends ever since.

Josh witnessed one of my most embarrassing moments. The first day of first grade, I couldn't find the bathroom and was too shy to ask the teacher. Finally, I couldn't hold it in any longer and had an accident right there on the classroom floor. I figured if I didn't say anything, no one would notice. No luck. A kid behind me yelled triumphantly, "Andy peed in his pants!" Everyone looked, saw the big damp stain on my pants and laughed. To this day, Josh swears he wasn't the one who blew my cover, but I'm not so sure.

We learned tennis, basketball, and baseball together. We weren't amazing athletes, but we were tough competitors and we had a lot of fun. I remember when we played in our first basketball league. The coach never let us have the ball, which really frustrated us. One day in practice, though, he passed it to me. It might have been an accident. I turned to Josh and said, "You have to feel this thing. I knew it was round, but I didn't think it was so rough." We thought that was hysterical, but the coach didn't. He continued benching us.

Josh and I spent every waking hour together. We both performed in school talent shows, though neither of us had any identifiable talent. We both had a crush on our fourth-grade teacher, Ms. Powell. We spent so much time together that friends mixed us up. They'd call me Josh and him Andy. If they saw Josh, they'd ask where I was, and if they saw me, they'd ask where Josh was.

The only time we were rivals was in competition, unless, of course, we were playing doubles in tennis. Josh was the only guy I didn't beat when I won that trophy at tennis camp. We tied. In second grade, he beat me in the finals of the school spelling bee. I will never misspell "invisible" again. Each of us had and have a lot of respect for the other, but that has never stopped us from wanting to beat the other's butt into the ground. Josh once broke both his feet in a college two-on-two basketball tournament, but he finished the game. Stupid, but tough. He used to tell me, "If you try zero percent of the time, you'll fail 100 percent of the time." He doesn't make or accept excuses. He makes me realize that I can do anything as long as I do my best.

Josh has never treated me differently because I have CF. When I coughed, he never asked if I was O.K. When I gasped for air, he didn't pity me. On the contrary, he pushed me to work harder. If I was losing a tennis match or basketball game, he'd urge me to rally and win. That meant a lot to me because when I was growing up, my family and doctors were obsessed with my health and always warned me not to overexert myself. Josh didn't pay any attention to what the doctors said. He saw me as a friend and a competitor, not some sick kid.

9

GROWING UP
IN A RUSH

Fall 1991 – Age 18

Josh and I attended fraternity rush at the University of Georgia and went from house to house to meet the brothers. We saw a lot of liquor in those two days. All the fraternities gave the same speech: "We have a nice house. We do well in academics. We are great in athletics." Blah, blah, blah.

The first house I visited was Alpha Epsilon Pi, which was supposed to be the "cool" Jewish fraternity. The brothers there urged me to join, and before I knew it, they gave me a pen to sign my bid. I was ready to do it until I remembered that I'd heard about another Jewish fraternity on campus. I asked the AEPi brothers and they laughed.

"Yeah, there's Tau Epsilon Phi, but you don't want to join them. They're a bunch of losers," a guy named Michael said with a snicker.

I usually give in pretty easily to peer pressure, but on that day, I didn't. I felt I should weigh all my options before making such an important decision. I told them I'd check out the other fraternity and if they were right, I'd be back. Michael quit snickering.

"C'mon, man. Just sign," he said, sliding the bid card closer to me. "Don't be a loser, man."

I thought, if this place is so great, why do they have to work so hard to convince me to join?

The next day I visited Tau Epsilon Phi. I got directions from a guy who said if I walked a half-mile down Baxter Street, I'd see the house. "How will I know which one it is?" I asked. He laughed and said, "You'll know it when you see it."

I walked a half-mile and didn't see the fraternity house. I did pass a decrepit home that looked like a Civil War relic waiting for the demolition crew. The columns on the porch were askew, and some bricks were missing from the façade. The windows were cracked. The roof looked like it was made of rocks and loose wire. In the back, I could see a basketball goal with a bent rim two feet too short. I noticed a lot of people in the yard and wondered why they were gathered at a condemned house. Then I saw three letters on the front: T-E-P.

The interior was a perfect match for the exterior. As I entered the house, I heard a girl squeal, "Was that a rat?" The floor looked like it hadn't been mopped since the 1930s, and some of the benches in the dining area didn't have legs. The pool table was missing several balls, but didn't lack cigarette or beer stains. The closets were all locked, but I could hear something rattling in one of them. On the bright side, I figured I'd found Jimmy Hoffa. The only redeeming feature was the ice machine. It made the clearest, freshest cubes of ice I'd ever seen.

After a lunch of rubbery steak, I met all the brothers. I was surprised to notice how nice they seemed. When I told them I was considering joining their rival, Alpha Epsilon Pi, I expected them to sneer and make crude remarks about them. But they didn't.

One of the brothers said, "TEP is great, but you have to choose which fraternity makes you happiest." That took a lot of pressure off me. For the first time since I'd walked onto the University of Georgia campus, I felt comfortable. I spent several hours there talking with them about standard guy stuff: women, sports, and cars.

Maybe TEP could be a home away from home for me. As I walked back to my dorm, I thought about which fraternity I should join. Would it be Alpha Epsilon Pi, "the coolest Jewish fraternity on campus," or would it be Tau Epsilon Phi, which had an amazing ice machine? Josh and I talked it over that night and again the next morning. We decided on TEP. It was predominately Jewish and the brothers were genuine - even if they weren't "the coolest" people in the world. Hey, I wasn't exactly the big man on campus either. We

chose a Jewish fraternity because we didn't have a lot
of Jewish friends in high school and we thought it
would be nice to meet people with similar back-
grounds. We returned to the TEP house to tell the
brothers. They grinned, slapped us on the back, and
shook our hands. We sat and chatted for several hours,
and I knew I'd made a good decision.

We arrived the next week for our first pledge meeting. After waiting a while, a guy finally came up to us
and screamed, "Sit down and shut up, you low-life
pledges!" "Oh my God," I thought, "What the heck is
going on?"

Pledging, we learned, was a humbling and occasion-
ally humiliating experience. Whatever the brothers told
us to do, we did. They didn't physically hurt us, but they
did devise lots of schemes to embarrass us and exasper-
ate us. We had to call each other by our pledge names.
Mine was "Cyrano." I wasn't too familiar with Cyrano
de Bergerac, but I'd seen "Roxanne" and I knew the
brothers were mocking my rather, uh, prominent nose,
one of my biggest insecurities. We had to carry the
brothers' books to class and memorize each one's hometown, major, and interests. We had to learn fraternity
trivia and stats about famous UGA football moments.

Sometimes I'd ask myself, "What's the point?" But I
didn't want to quit, though the brothers would have
understood, I think. On our pledge sheets, we had to
disclose any illnesses and an emergency contact, so they
knew I had CF. They often asked if I was overburdened

by the pledge demands and told me it was O.K. to miss a pledge meeting if I had to. I wasn't used to people giving me an "out" because of CF. I would not allow that to be an option. I was going to be a brother in Tau Epsilon Phi by doing everything my fellow pledges did. Furthermore, I was building friendships with my pledge brothers. Strong friendships.

10

CHANGING MY OUTLOOK

Fall 1991 – Age 18

Not long after I became a TEP pledge, a bunch of pledge brothers and I went to lunch at the cafeteria. Though I was among guys who I thought should be my friends, I was miserable. Everyone was ridiculing me.

At the time, I had a nondescript haircut and my hair was perpetually out of control. My shirts were about two sizes too small, when oversized clothing was fashionable. I never bought new clothes – that was my mom's department. I still wore the blue jeans she bought me from Kmart. On my feet was a ratty pair of gray tennis shoes I'd had since my sophomore year of high school. I was no fashion plate. I knew this, but I really didn't think much about it until these guys began taunting my appearance.

I didn't defend myself because I was afraid that the only way I could compensate for any personal shortcomings was to do whatever my pledge brothers asked. Then they'd hang out with me. I always felt that because of CF, I'd have to go the extra mile to make friends. I presumed it was tough on them because I was, after all, so different.

So I listened to the guys tease me about my geeky wardrobe and non-existent love life. It wasn't the first time they'd said those things. I had slowly grown used to it. This day, though, one of my pledge brothers, Aaron, said something that cut me to the core: "Andy, man, the only reason why people hang out with you is that you have a car and you drive them everywhere." I'd driven everyone to the cafeteria that afternoon, in fact. Secretly, I was afraid that what he said was true. I was so upset that I called him an asshole and stormed out of the cafeteria. Let them find their own way home.

I drove back to the dorm, fell on my bed, and cried. Was Aaron right? Was I so desperate for "friends" that I was willing to sacrifice my self-esteem? Why did people make fun of me? And why didn't Josh stand up for me? He's known me forever and he never cared how I dressed. I guess, like me, he was afraid of our friends' opinions. When you get to college, you feel a need to fit in – even when fitting in means not coming to your best friend's rescue.

Later that day, Josh and another brother came by to see me. I kept my face in the pillow. The phone rang. It was Aaron. I refused to talk to him, but he said something to Josh, and Josh put the phone next to my ear.

"Dude," Aaron said, "I'm sorry, but it's the truth."

"You're an asshole!" I yelled and hung up on him.

A couple hours later, there was a knock at my door. I didn't want to answer it, but the knocking didn't stop. I wiped the tears from my face and opened the door. It was Aaron.

"What?" I asked, ready to shut the door in his obnoxious face.

"Look, dude, I'm just trying to help you out," he said. "You obviously lack self-esteem. You can't say 'no' to anyone. You don't know how to dress. You don't know how to talk to girls. You don't –"

"O.K.," I interrupted him. "I get the point. Why don't you help me then?"

Aaron considered that for a second and pounced on the idea. "Well, O.K., but you have to be willing to make some drastic changes."

I wondered what those would be. I had no social life, no girlfriend, and no self-esteem. Basically, I had nothing to lose. "I'll do it," I said. "Let's get started."

That night, Aaron went through my closet item by item. He said he'd remove everything I had that was not cool. He removed all my tee shirts, saying, "They make you look like a tool." A tool being synonomous with a dweeb or a geek. He also ditched my caps, my white underwear, my white socks, my tennis shoes, every pair of shorts I owned, all my collared shirts, and my sports memorabilia. Never wear stuff with sports logos, he warned, and never wear plain white socks. I didn't know where he got these rules or if they even made sense, but I just nodded. By the time he was done, I had one T-shirt, a few pairs of cotton boxers, a plain baseball cap, a pair of ripped-up khaki shorts, and a pair of running shoes.

Aaron also told me that if I wanted a girlfriend, I'd need to toss my sports posters and bathing suit calendars. "The calendar pictures intimidate girls, and they think sports posters are immature," he said. Well, whatever. I asked if I could at least keep Miss March. Aaron laughed and shook his head. I told him I was a big Braves fan, but he reminded me that if I wanted a girlfriend, I'd have to make some sacrifices. So there went my Braves tee shirts.

He also suggested I change my attitude and style: Keep your head up and make eye contact with girls. "Don't be afraid to talk to a girl," he said. "If she doesn't like you, forget about her. Move on. Nobody is better than you." I never forgot that. He also told me to stop telling so many stupid jokes because they made me sound like a moron. Well, whatever. But honestly, I'd never be cured of that habit. I learned to make people laugh when I was little. I found that jokes protected me from the serious discussions about cystic fibrosis. A way to lighten the mood.

Aaron also told me to stand up for myself and say "no" now and then. "The most important thing," he concluded, "is to always—"

"I know, I know," I said. "Always be myself."

He stared at me like I had three eyes. "Heck, no. What are you, an idiot?"

I think he was kidding. At least, I hope so.

The next day, Aaron and I went to the mall for my "makeover." At the mall, I tried on more clothes than Claudia Schiffer on a fashion shoot. Some of the things he liked, I never would have bought.

"Aaron, I think these jeans are too tight. I can't feel things I should be able to feel."

"That means they're perfect," he said with a nod. "We'll take them."

We bought three short-sleeved shirts with collars, two pairs of khakis, a green wool cap, two long-sleeved collared shirts, two pairs of jeans, a couple of pairs of nice socks, and a bottle of Obsession cologne. When my mom got the bill a month later, she asked me if the credit card had been stolen. I hadn't spent that much money in a mall in all my 18 years. I told her the truth, but by the time she was done scolding me for spending three hundred dollars, I was wishing I'd lied. It was the first time I'd bought clothes without my mother's help. It was also one of the first times that someone at school had done something nice for me and expected nothing in return.

Spending time at the mall made me think about the dream I'd been having for years, the one where I was hiding under a clothes rack in a mall and a friendly girl asked me if I needed help. Maybe she wanted to help me change my wardrobe, my image, and my attitude.

Could that be it?

That night I made my debut at a TEP house party. I strolled in wearing hiking boots, a new pair of jeans, a wool cap and a beige long-sleeve collared shirt over a T-shirt. The scent of Obsession floated through the air. I got looks – not the same kind of looks as when I wheeled my therapy machine into the dorm. Rather, I got smiles and nods.

Someone laughed and asked if I was Aaron's protégé. I took it as a compliment because if I was going to take after someone, Aaron wasn't a bad choice. When Josh saw me, he said, "You're dressed like the ultimate fraternity guy. We're going to have to call you 'Fraternity Lipman.'" That eventually got shortened to "Flip," which my fraternity brothers call me to this day. It's a heck of a lot better than "Cyrano."

Aaron and I became close friends after our shopping excursion. I liked him because he took a real interest in me and because he wasn't bothered by the fact that I had CF. When people would find out that I had CF and then get that polite, concerned look on their faces, Aaron would interject, "Yeah, he can't breathe or anything. I think he's missing a lung. Does anyone see it? I hope he didn't lose it in the Jello again." When I'd be doubled over with a coughing attack, other people might nervously ask if I was O.K. Aaron would ask me if he should call the coroner.

That might sound cruel, but it was funny to me. I'd lived for so long with CF and dire reports about my health and life expectancy that it was a relief to hear someone joke about it. I was very much alive. When Aaron cracked jokes about CF, I'd think, "Hey, this isn't so bad. I can laugh at it. And I can beat it."

I remember one time when I was returning to my dorm after class. I heard a familiar sound coming from my room. I opened the door and there was Aaron in my therapy vest as the machine was cranking away, thumping his chest. He was bright red and laughing. He claimed he'd lost a lung and thought my machine might help. I couldn't help laughing either. Who would have thought that something as essential to my health as a no-nonsense therapy machine could be a hilarious gag when Aaron put it on? Not only was it funny, but it made me feel good to see someone else wear the vest for once. I didn't feel so different anymore.

Aaron helped transform my attitude about CF. I had been so secretive about it for fear that people would think I was odd or sick, but my friendship with him made me realize someone could like me for me. He didn't care about the fact that I had CF any more than he cared that I was from Atlanta or that I was a Braves fan. It was one fact about me, but it didn't define me. At least, it didn't define me any more than I was willing to let it. That was an important lesson, but unfortunately, it was one that I forgot all too quickly.

11

RUDE AWAKENING

Spring 1993 – Age 19

By my sophomore year, everything began to come together. I felt comfortable on the campus and knew lots of guys and girls. I moved out of the dorm and into the TEP fraternity house. My room really felt like home. I hung a bikini calendar on the wall behind my dusty couch. I knew Aaron had said not to have bikini calendars, but I'd already changed my wardrobe, and there was just something about Miss October. I had to duck to get into the room because my loft was so low, but it was comfortable and more importantly, it was mine. It was a loft decorated with quotes – maybe you'd call it graffiti – from brothers who lived there back in the early '80s. My favorite was "Reach for the moon. Even if you miss, you'll still be among the stars." My heater worked only half the time so the winter was tough to handle, but spring was now upon us.

My goal that year was to find a girlfriend. It was the only thing that seemed to be missing from my life. When I was younger, I dreamt of one girl, the girl who approached me when I was hiding under the clothes rack. She asked if I needed help. Was she the one I'd meet here? She was very pretty with brown hair and warm, friendly brown eyes. After I told her I didn't need help, she'd then disappear into the store, and I'd wake up. That was probably the closest thing I ever had to a girl being interested in my well-being.

Not that there weren't great girls at UGA. I had a major crush on a fraternity brother's girlfriend, Helayne. When I was a freshman, I used to write her poetry, and when she sprained her ankle during a softball game, I took her a teddy bear. In addition to being beautiful – brown eyes, tanned skin, and a cheerleader's athletic body – she was funny, sweet, and easy to talk to. Basically, all she was missing was a halo. I'd fantasize about rescuing her from kidnappers or saving her life and winning her admiration, gratitude, and eternal love. It sounds a little corny, but I wanted to be the hero. I could dream, couldn't I?

Things were going great, I thought, until one late night in the fraternity house. It was about 2:30 a.m.; a bunch of us were watching a movie. I was finishing my therapy. The door was ajar, which was no big deal. My fraternity brothers were all used to the machine. They knew it sounded like a jet during takeoff. They'd seen me wear the therapy vest and breathe the aerosols from the nebulizer. That's why I was able to relax my self-conscious sentiments. They knew I had CF and they accepted me for that.

As I was doing therapy, Sally*, another girl who I was interested in and one I thought liked me, peeked in the room. She saw me and a wave of what I took to be horror and disgust raced across her pretty face. I froze. "I am leaving! Bye!" I could hear her say. She didn't say good-bye to me. Was I that revolting? Did I look like an alien with all sorts of freakish tubes attached to its body?

I thought people accepted me. I thought people knew me as Andy, not some freak. I was always going to have to use this machine and always have to take medication and always disgust women. I ripped off the vest and pulled the nebulizer from my mouth. "Get out," I yelled. "Everyone get out!" I know it seemed that I now had so much confidence. After all, I had changed my wardrobe. I had made so many new friends. But it was like the time I read the encyclopedia article. I thought everything was going well, but deep down, I was still insecure. It was only a matter of time before that one issue was going to present itself and change everything.

One of my fraternity brothers asked, "What? What is it?" But I couldn't tell him.

"I have to go to bed," I yelled. "I'm tired."

I slammed the door shut and locked it. I pounded on it until my fist was sore. I hated this stupid machine. I hated this stupid disease. I hated myself. I hated my parents for giving it to me. I hated them all. Why did I hate everyone? I didn't know. I just felt if one person thought I was different because of my CF, then everyone would think I was a freak. So many insecurities came to the forefront. Were people friends with me because they liked me or because they pitied me? Was I ever going to meet a girl who thought of me as a man? Would I always be thought of as a case study? College is such a tough time. It's your first opportunity to be on your own. You are judged by your peers. Some people are prepared for that. I suppose I wasn't ready to be judged.

I threw the vest on the floor and kicked the machine. Why do they have to be so ignorant? I wanted to die. God, just kill me already. I started to cry and jammed my pillow on top of my head. "Damnit. I am a loser." I grabbed at my hair and pulled it out, strand by strand. "I'll always be a loser and it's all because of CF." I didn't want to face the people who thought of me as a freak. Everyone pretended to like me, but they didn't. They just felt sorry for me. God must have hated me. He must really have hated me to give me CF.

12

WHY ME?

Spring 1993 – Age 19

The next morning, I woke up with a sick feeling, remembering what had happened the night before. Why bother with breakfast? I didn't want anyone to see me. Girls thought I was grotesque, and my friends probably thought so too. That's why they were nice to me. They felt sorry for me because I have CF. I should have known it all along. All I had to do was remember the pledge football game from a few months ago.

It was the annual contest between our pledges and our arch rivals, Alpha Epsilon Pi. It was my chance to show my fraternity brothers and fellow pledges what I could do athletically, and it was a chance to impress the girls who'd be watching. I was eager to play, but a little puzzled. During the weeks we were practicing, the coaches kept asking me, "Do you need to take a break?," "Are you okay?," and "Are you sure you can do these exercises?" Of course I was sure. I went to practice every day and memorized the plays. I worked on my defense. I worked on my offense. Each night before I fell asleep I pictured myself catching the winning touchdown. My teammates would cheer and carry me off the field; the girls would all want me, and the guys would all want to be my friend.

The day of the game, the coaches told me I wouldn't be starting. I was a little upset by that, but it would be O.K. It's not who starts that matters – it's who finishes. As the game progressed, my excitement began to wane. I wanted to play already. By the fourth quarter, our team was down by two touchdowns. I might not have been the hero, but at least I'd get to play, I thought. I put myself in the coaches' line of vision, figuring they couldn't possibly miss me. But they wouldn't look at me. The final seconds ran down and our team lost.

Why didn't they put me in? I asked a coach. He told me: "We didn't want you to get hurt. The fraternity can't risk a lawsuit." That stung. It was obvious that I was being treated differently because I had CF. I was sick of standing on the sidelines. I wanted to participate with everyone else. Wasn't that obvious? I never asked to be treated differently because of CF or expected anyone to give me a special break. It was as if my mom had written another note.

I woke to a knock on the door. My clock said 6 p.m.

"Let's go out," Josh hollered.

"Nah," I said. "I don't feel well. I'm tired." I didn't

want to see his face or anyone else's, for that matter.

"C'mon, man. We'll be back in a few hours and then you can go back to bed."

"No thanks. I don't feel well. Leave me alone."

I faked a coughing spasm.

"Alright man, fine. Feel better. Talk to you later."

I knew CF was good for something – making people feel sorry for me. I fell back asleep, only to be awakened four hours later by another knock.

"Dude, you home?" my fraternity brother Greg asked. "Let's go, man. The party's starting."

I didn't answer.

"C'mon man, let's go. Let's meet some chicks."

Just what I needed to do. They could all sit together and giggle about the hideous sight of a guy they thought was normally connected to something that looked like life support. Obviously, if one girl knew, everyone knew. They were probably discussing it now. I bet they were trying to figure out how long I'd live. No wonder no one wanted to go out with me. I could hear Greg knock again and then heard his footsteps grow softer until they disappeared.

I realized I hadn't eaten in nearly 24 hours. But I didn't want to go to the kitchen because then everyone would ask where I'd been and why I was hiding out. The last thing I wanted to do was run into the girl whose face contorted in disgust when she saw me during therapy. I wasn't going to use it that night, I decided. I didn't want anyone to hear it running. The sound wasn't easy to miss or ignore.

I remember my freshman year in the dorm when I'd use the machine. My neighbors would pound on the wall because it was so loud. I didn't want to tell them the machine was helping to keep me alive because I had a life-threatening genetic illness. I didn't want their pity. I did my part to look normal. I lied. I hid the machine in my closet. But still, people knew. And still, they stared with a mix of curiosity and, I think, pity.

By 3:30 a.m. the band finally called it quits. The voices in the hall quieted and the only sound I could hear was the steady chirp of the crickets. I went to the bathroom for the first time since Friday. I was hungry, but I decided to wait until morning to eat. No one would be sober enough to be up before noon. At 10 a.m. Sunday morning, I tiptoed out of the house and headed to Shoney's. I bought a 12-inch strawberry pie and wolfed it down. I ate nothing else and skipped my therapy again. I couldn't remember the last time I didn't do my therapy. Doing it every day was part of my routine, like taking a shower or brushing my teeth. It was one of the only parts of my daily life that reminded me I had CF. Skipping therapy would make me feel like everyone else though. I'd get an extra 40 minutes back in my life each day.

After two days without therapy, though, I was having trouble breathing. Every time I inhaled, I heard a rattle in my chest. My cough, which was rare, had become deep and hacking, the way hard-core smokers' coughs sound. I realized I had also skipped my medication all weekend. I didn't take my vitamins or antibiotics. Because I didn't eat, I didn't take my Pancrease, which helps my pancreas digest fatty foods. I decided to take my medication and do my therapy on Monday.

When I woke up that morning, I couldn't stop coughing. My chest was throbbing and my throat was hoarse. I felt like I had heaved up my guts and couldn't stop. I was coughing so badly I couldn't walk to class. I made my way outside, but I had to stop and bend over because the coughing spasms made it impossible to stand. I was drained. I decided to skip my classes and rest. I knew I could always tell my instructors I had CF; they'd surely feel sorry for me, combating a life-threatening illness.

That night I did my therapy, thinking I'd feel better. I didn't. I'd never felt worse.

The next day, I skipped classes again. I still felt congested and my sides ached from coughing. But I thought I could play basketball. I realized how wrong I was. I began coughing up chunks of phlegm. It was a light green color, which scared me because my doctors had warned me that if it was anything but clear, I had an infection. I kept coughing. My chest was pounding. My teammates, the guys who are supposed to be my "friends," asked me if I was going through puberty because my voice was so hoarse.

I couldn't stand it anymore. I yelled two words I never thought I'd say: "I quit!" I had never felt like

quitting before. Even when I tried out for the fraternity
softball team as a freshman and the captain told me I
probably wouldn't displace any of the returning seniors
for a spot on the team, I didn't quit. I didn't make the
team, but I did the best I could. Quitting was new to
me. It was not really my fault, though. Didn't my doctors say that as CF patients get older, their bodies dete-
riorate? This was normal.

My coughing worsened and my stamina decreased.
I knew I should have seen a doctor, but why bother?
Why pay good money to hear the inevitable, that my
days were numbered? I had to see a doctor, though, if
only because I went twice a year to a CF specialist in
North Carolina, Thomas Boat. Dr. Boat was a nice guy,
but that didn't mean I wanted to go or tell him anything
about my life. Maybe that's because I couldn't shake
the memory of my first visit to his office.

I was 15 and went with my parents to the University
of North Carolina Children's Hospital. I was nervous
to begin with, and being subjected to a virtual parade
of sick, dying, and helpless children terrified me. I saw
a little boy a few years younger than me in a wheelchair
in the corner of the waiting room. His eyes were glassy
and barely open, set deep in a pale face. Tubes were
connected to his frail arms. He coughed continuously
and looked like he was in pain.

I was in the pulmonary department when someone
said that this little boy had cystic fibrosis. I'd seen por-
tions of Alex's movie on television and browsed

through the CF encyclopedia article, but this was different. I couldn't just turn off the television or close the book and live my life. This was another person, someone who was suffering, someone with the same genetic disorder I had. I wondered how long he would live and if he even wanted to live. Then I asked the same questions about myself. How long did I have to live? Would I end up a shadow of myself, confined to a wheelchair, a burden on my parents and a pitiful sight to others?

Each time I returned to the hospital, I remembered that boy and remembered that all I ever wanted to do when I visited Dr. Boat was to get out as quickly as possible. On this visit, it was obvious that something was wrong. My phlegm was bright green and I was coughing, gasping, and wheezing. Yet I refused to believe I wasn't well.

When I took the pulmonary function test, I expected my breathing capacity to be as impressive as it always was. Usually the test administrator would examine my results and say, "Wow! You have CF? No way." This time, though, she didn't say anything as she made a notation on my chart. I asked for another chance, but I did even worse. The third time was my worst score. I was blowing as hard as I could into the tube, but it didn't seem to be helping. I felt light-headed and feared I'd pass out. My God, I'm a sophomore in college. My concerns should be calculus homework or weekend social plans. Not death! A nurse examined me and asked the same questions she always did. I lied.

I knew if I admitted anything, they'd haul my butt into the hospital, where I'd probably die. If I gave the usual answers, maybe they'd allow me to go home.

"Are you spitting up phlegm?"

"Uh, not really."

"When you do, what color is it?"

"Usually clear."

"Nothing green or yellow?"

"Nope."

"Are you coughing a lot?"

"No, just the usual amount."

She looked at me suspiciously.

"Do you feel pain in your chest when you cough?"

God, yes. "No."

While I was waiting with my mom and little sister Emily for my X-rays to be processed, I imagined what Dr. Boat would say: "Andy, I'm very disappointed in you. You need to take better care of yourself. See you in a few months."

I wished my dad were there. He usually came with us, but he was called away on a business meeting. He would know what to do if he was here.

When Dr. Boat entered the room, I knew something was wrong. Unlike all the other times I'd seen him, he seemed reluctant to speak to us. "Well," he said, "I looked at Andy's X-rays, and we need to make some changes immediately before the bacteria in his lungs spreads."

He looked at me. "Your health isn't as good as it

was the last time we met."

No kidding.

"I'm not sure why."

I wasn't going to volunteer any information.

"The X-rays show a definite inflammation in Andy's lungs," he said, turning to my mom. "We'll have to do a sputum culture to see if it's pseudomonas."

My mother's eyes darted to Dr. Boat's face. "Pseudomonas? Do you think it's that?"

"All I'm saying is it's a possibility," he said calmly, "and we need to investigate to see if that's what it is."

I'd heard the word "pseudomonas" mentioned before in my parents' conversations with doctors, but I never knew what it was. Judging from my mom's reaction, it was serious.

Dr. Boat scanned my chart. "Your pulmonary function scores are down considerably from last time. We're going to have to change some of your medicines. Let's see...are you getting a lot of exercise?"

What was I going to say? That I lie in my bed for 48 hours at a time, sometimes without eating a thing? Oh, and I don't do my therapy or take many of my medications anymore. Of course I couldn't tell him that. He'd freak out. My mom would freak out. She'd yank me out of Georgia.

"Oh, yeah, I play basketball. Tennis. Softball. And football. Every sport. Never felt in better shape. Yeah, I do my therapy every day. Always take my medication."

I would've said I played Australian Rules football if

it would rip that suspicious look off Dr. Boat's face. I knew he didn't believe me. In my brain, a chorus played, "I'm scared I'm going to die. I'm scared I'm going to die. I'm scared I'm going to die." Could my mom hear it? I looked at her, hoping she'd reassure me, but she didn't say anything. Tears filled my eyes and trickled down my cheeks.

"I think he's really scared, Dr. Boat. Can you tell him he will get better?"

Gee, thanks Mom. That's what you call support?

Dr. Boat's face softened a little. "Andy, we're going to do everything to get to the bottom of this and get you back on track," he said. "If you take care of yourself, you should be fine."

How reassuring. Why not measure me now for the casket? What's with the "should" and "could"? It sounded like he knew something I didn't, and that could only be something bad. I'm going to die. I am truly a failure.

Dr. Boat prescribed some strong antibiotics and an inhaler. Just what I needed. Something else to make me look like a freak. He said he wanted to see me again soon, but I knew the next time he'd see me, it would be for an autopsy. The pessimism in the room crushed my chest. No wonder I had a hard time breathing.

We got in the car for the long ride home. My mom told me I'd be O.K. "We'll get through this," she said. I could sense that she was frightened, and I thought she was putting on a front so that I wouldn't be more

scared than I already was. I remembered the encyclopedia article that said I'd be dead by 25 and the CF movie
with the sad ending. They were the reality. I just hadn't
accepted it until now.

"Andy, it's O.K.," my mom said again. Her eyes
were framed in the rear-view mirror. "Just take better
care of yourself. Do your therapy twice a day. Take the
new medications Dr. Boat prescribed. Things will get
better. You'll see."

No they won't, I thought. I was going to die. "I hate
you. I hate everyone. Leave me alone."

She pulled into the McDonald's parking lot. Emily
was clamoring for McNuggets.

"We'll talk over lunch," my mom said.

"I'm staying in the car."

"Don't be selfish. Your sister needs to eat."

And I guess that's when I lost it. "Me, selfish? You
must be kidding. I'm the one who's sacrificing my life
to some stupid disease."

Emily opened the car door and was skipping toward
the restaurant door, waving to us to hurry up. I didn't
move. My mother began to cry.

"Please, Andy. You can get through this. This isn't
easy for me, either."

I started crying too. The sight of my mom in tears
always does that to me. But I refused to feel sorry for
her. She wasn't the one who was suffering.

"I don't care if I die," I sobbed. "You don't care
either. Dad doesn't care; he's not even here."

I knew I was hurting her, but I wanted to.

"I do care, and so does Dad." Her eyes met mine with a hard glance. "Stop feeling sorry for yourself. It will do you no good. Let's eat."

"I don't want to eat. I don't need to eat. I'll die faster if I don't eat."

My mother sighed in exasperation. "Andy, please. I can't take this any more. You're not being fair to me."

"Fair to you?" I screeched. "You think this is fair to me? You gave me this stupid disease! How do you think I feel? Just leave me alone! Let me die in peace!"

My mother let out a wrenching cry that cut into my heart. Great, heaving sobs made her shoulders shake, and her head was bowed in grief. I'd never seen her weep like that before. Tears dripped onto her blouse, leaving little opaque circles. I knew what I said hurt her more than I could fathom. No doubt she did blame herself for the fact that her only son had CF. No doubt she spent many nights fearing exactly what I feared, but put on a brave face so I would be fearless.

I wanted to tell her I was sorry. I wanted her to hold me and rock me like she did when I was little and had skinned my knee. I wanted to beg her to make everything better, like she always used to do with a Band-Aid and a kiss. I couldn't do it though. I still clung to the anger I felt in Dr. Boat's office when she didn't leap to my defense. I was too preoccupied with my own sad state of affairs to give much thought to how I'd wronged anyone else.

After lunch, we drove back to Georgia in silence. I thought about my body's steady deterioration. I could be dead before I graduate from college. I didn't want to go back to school anyway. My "friends" already thought I was a loser. I hadn't been to class in weeks. I knew I was failing calculus. I hated my life and I hated myself.

13

FADING AWAY

Winter 1993 – Age 20

When I got back to school, I easily slid into my new routine – I went straight to bed. I was obsessed by thoughts of death and dying. I couldn't think about anything else. When I managed to sleep, it was never for long. Coughing spasms would wake me repeatedly during the night. I'd sit in the dark hacking up huge chunks of phlegm. I stopped answering the phone and the door. This no longer seemed strange to me. I wanted to be left alone to die. I wanted people to feel guilty about how they treated me.

I especially wanted Josh to feel that way. Josh was the one person I felt I could always count on and always confide in. Lately, however, I'd felt our friendship slipping away. Instead of spending time with me, he was busy with his new girlfriend. To make matters worse, my fraternity brothers had been bragging that since Josh began working out, he was irresistible to women. In most instances I'd be happy for Josh, but since I wasn't happy with myself, I didn't want to hear that my best friend was thriving.

I remembered one evening I was watching a video with a girl named Amy who I thought really liked me. She knew I had CF and she didn't seem to care, which was a great sign as far as I was concerned. As we watched the movie, she asked if I knew when Josh would be home. Was he seeing anyone? Did I think he'd go out with her? I was crushed. She obviously wasn't hanging out with me because she was interested in me. I remembered when Josh and I were so alike that people used to mix us up. When had he become a stud and I become a dud?

I stopped going to parties. A couple times I thought about showing my face, but when I'd grip the door-knob, I'd hear voices in the hall and then I'd lose my nerve. I'd creep back to my couch and put a pillow over my head. I feared people would see me and remember what a freak I was. The more time I spent in my room, the harder it became to leave. I felt more and more isolated and didn't know how to break away. Honestly, I wasn't sure I wanted to. This went on for a little less than a year.

At night I'd listen to Jimmy Buffet's "Feeding Frenzy," hoping his laid-back lyrics would inspire me. I rented inspiring sports videos like "The Karate Kid" and "Rocky" with the same hope. They didn't work either. All they did was remind me of how far I'd sunk after being such an accomplished athlete. The days dragged on. I felt less than alive. I knew something was desperately wrong. I needed to talk to someone, but felt there was no one who I could confide in. When I was younger I used to vent to my dog, Howard, but he had died a month after I left for college. I considered going to a psychiatrist, but my only means of payment was with my parents' credit card. As soon as they saw the bill, they would have known I was in a crisis. As much as I needed help, I didn't want to admit any weakness. I felt that it would have only confirmed to them that I should never have gone away to school because, clearly, I couldn't take care of myself.

I spiraled into a deep depression, and I lost the will to fight it. I began skipping therapy again. The drugs that Dr. Boat prescribed sat on my dresser. I didn't take them. I talked to almost no one. When my mom called, I'd quickly wrap up conversations by telling her I was just getting ready to go out with friends. That way we couldn't talk for more than a few minutes and she wouldn't be able to sense that something was wrong. I knew I couldn't have talked to her for long without sobbing for help. I hid in my room each weekend and told my friends I was going home because I didn't feel well. I never went to the grocery store or out to eat...I basically starved myself. I even began parking my car blocks from the fraternity house so no one would know I was home.

Since I'd alienated my old group of friends, I fell into a different crowd. I spent a lot of time with a couple of guys named Russ* and Stan*. Stan was not happy with the fraternity because everyone accused him of stealing. "I knew that feeling of being treated like an outsider," I said with a nod. Russ had problems, too. He said his parents had all but abandoned him. We'd talk about suicide. He said he'd like to climb to the top seats of the football stadium and hurl himself over the side. The way he described it, I could imagine it. I thought I could die that way too.

At night my brain was crammed with thoughts of death. I envisioned buying a gun and blowing my brains out. Or buying yards of strong rope, tying a noose, and hanging myself. The next morning Josh would come in and find my lifeless body hanging from the ceiling in the bathroom. He'd be overcome with grief and remorse. I wanted him to hate himself as much as I hated myself. I thought about death so much that I was no longer scared of it. It would have come almost as a relief.

My dreams were grim, with the exception of a single recurring one. I continued to dream about the girl in the mall. She kept asking me if I needed help. No, I told her. I didn't need her help. When I said that, she'd vanish. But she was persistent. She returned night after night, always politely asking if I needed help. My answer was not honest, but it never changed. No, I told her. I didn't need her help.

I slept fitfully. While the rest of the fraternity brothers snored and dreamed, I was awake. I'd cough myself
out of sleep and heave up chunks of viscous phlegm.
Night after night, I'd wake in a cold sweat, which
would mix with my tears of pain and the globs of
mucous my body produced. I couldn't even sleep in my
loft bed anymore. I slept on the sofa because I knew I
would have to stumble to the shower to clean myself
off. As I fumbled with the faucets and rinsed the filth
from my increasingly emaciated body, I plotted as best
I could. How could I get a gun? When and where would
I kill myself? Who would really care if I were dead?

I continued to live in the fraternity house, but I had
nothing to do with my brothers. They eventually
stopped inviting me to parties and games. Instead, they
stared at me openly the way I always thought people
stared at me secretly. They appeared to be horrified,
disgusted, confused, and even bored by me. It was obvious to me that they had no idea what was happening to
my body or my brain and if they had, they could've
cared less.

14

THE FINAL CRY

Winter 1993 – Age 20

I couldn't find my accounting textbook. Seeing that I'd been skipping classes for weeks, I thought I'd misplaced it. I checked my backpack, the backseat of my car, my desk, and under my bed. I didn't know where else it could be. I asked Stan and Russ if they'd seen it. Both said no. So I went to the bookstore to buy another copy. Then I remembered a brief conversation I had with them earlier that day. It stopped me cold. Russ had mentioned that he and Stan had sold back their textbooks after final exams.

I asked an employee at the bookstore if I could look at the accounting books that had been returned that day. Sure enough, there was an accounting book from my class, and it had my notes in it. I asked who sold it back, and they showed me Stan's signature on the receipt. Not only was he a thief, but he was a liar. I felt betrayed and angry. I had trusted him and stood up for him when others accused him of stealing, and this was how he repaid me. When I got back to the fraternity house, I confronted, and told him I'd seen his signature on the receipt at the bookstore. Despite that evidence, he denied selling back my book. He said he'd found the book in his room and assumed it was his. I knew that book had never left my room.

I tried to have Stan removed from the fraternity, which requires a 75% vote from the chapter's members. But I couldn't get enough votes. In other words, despite hard evidence that Stan was a thief and a liar, my fraternity brothers sided with him rather than with me. That really hurt. Despite what they said about being friends forever, they made it clear that I was only being tolerated, nothing more. It didn't matter that I was the person who had clearly been wronged. I saw Stan every day, and though we didn't hang out anymore, he acted like nothing had happened. For some reason, I felt like I had done something wrong in demanding that he be removed from TEP.

I had lost sight of who I was and what mattered to me. I really had no idea any longer what purpose I had, if any. I wasn't enjoying college. I was surviving it and struggling through each day. I found things coming out of my mouth that I never thought I'd say and that would have been - before this despair - unthinkable for me to utter.

One fraternity brother, Bert, was telling me how difficult it was for him to handle work and school. He told me, "You're spoiled. Your parents are loaded. You won't ever have to work a day in your life." None of that was true, and the "old me" would have told him so. Instead, I bitterly replied, "Yeah, well, at least you'll be alive in 10 years." There was absolutely nothing he could say in response, and I was glad. I deserved the pity. After all, I was dying. I'd gladly work 24 hours a day for the rest of my life in exchange for a life free from a CF death sentence.

Another time I was watching my pledge brothers play basketball. I spotted Brad*, who was having a tough time in classes. He was also having a tough time on the court. Instead of passing the ball to his teammates, he kept shooting it himself, which is not good strategy or team etiquette. I was in a foul mood, so I yelled, "You know the rules, Brad. No pass, no play" – which is what they tell student athletes with foul grades. He stopped cold on the court and his face flushed with shame. He glared at me.

"Asshole," he said and walked away.

The other players looked at me and shook their heads. "You know he's not doing well this quarter," one said. "How could you say that?" someone else added.

My grades were nothing to impress anyone. I'd missed weeks of class and didn't care too much. I had lost interest in studying, excelling, and learning. I was merely going through the motions of being a student.

The prior spring, I had to get a ride to see my calculus professor because I was too weak to walk. I told the instructor how sick I'd been – wasn't it obvious from looking at me? – and how weak I was. I cried and embellished my story to make myself even more pitiful.

She seemed sympathetic and told me that if I did well on the final, she'd take my illness into account. What a relief. She wouldn't be able to live with herself if she failed someone who was dying. She'd give me a C out of pity. One less thing to worry about.

When I got my grades for that quarter, my jaw dropped. I had two Cs in composition classes and an F in calculus. I had never failed a class in my life. What was I going to tell my parents?

My father was angry, so I wisely never told him how many classes I'd skipped, how little I'd studied, and how little I cared about anything. I explained that I'd always had a hard time with math and I was sick a lot. He looked disappointed, but all he said was to try harder next quarter.

I didn't though. The next quarter was just like the last one. I skipped class. Often I didn't have the stamina to drag myself to class. I stayed in my room with the lights off while fraternity parties downstairs rocked the house. It was obvious that these former "friends" had pegged me as a loser, an outcast. I began to hear what people said when they thought I'd gone home for the weekend. "Do you think Andy's gay?" they'd ask. "I don't know," someone else said. No matter how many times they said such things, it still hurt. Every time I felt wounded. I'd jam my pillow over my head and cry like it was the first time I'd heard it.

Now it was almost the end of winter quarter my junior year. Things hadn't changed for the better. A guy I knew told me he knew what I could do to feel better. "You need to try pot," he said. That was something I never would have considered when I was confident about my health, my athletic ability, and my "friends." Things were different now. I had nothing to lose because I was going to die anyway. Why not try it? He said he'd just bought a new stash and would be glad to share it with me the next night.

Though I knew nothing would change my mind, I called Aunt Susie that night to ask her if marijuana could hurt me. There was silence on the end of the line, then a long pause.

"Andy," she said, "don't be stupid. It could kill you. Promise me you won't do it."

"O.K., I promise," I said, just like that. I knew I was lying to someone who loved me. But I didn't care.

15

THE BASKETBALL GAME

Winter 1993 – Age 20

I woke up at noon on a Monday. This week was like each preceding one. There was nothing to look forward to. I planned to skip classes again, like every week. I'd spent the weekend hidden in my room crying and feeling sorry for myself, nourished only by a Shoney's strawberry pie. I pulled myself out of bed, showered, dressed, and made my way outside into the chilly winter afternoon. The wind was so strong I had to go back in and grab a heavier coat.

Then I saw him. It was the guy from the day before who had offered to share his pot with me. He was sitting in his car at the curb by the fraternity house. He waved to me to come over.

"Hey," he said, "I've got something to show you." He fumbled in the backseat and pulled out a bag of marijuana. I tried to look blasé, as though I'd seen pot before, but the truth was, I'd never seen marijuana up close.

"You excited about tonight?" he asked.

"Yeah, I guess."

"Good. It'll be cool. See you later."

I wandered over to the couch next to the basketball court near the fraternity house. I should have been in economics class, but I didn't want to go. I'd been to that class only once in the past three weeks. I was afraid the instructor would notice my absence – or, in this case, my presence. Instead, I sat bundled up on the couch. I had nowhere to go and didn't care.

A group of fraternity brothers came out of the house with a basketball and began to shoot baskets. It was a chilly day for a game, nearly 50 degrees, but at TEP the weather was always good enough for a game of 3-on-3. I envied their stamina and grace and remembered sadly how it felt to aim a jump shot and have perfect confidence that the ball would cleanly swish through the net.

"Ouch! I'm out!" someone yelled and interrupted my reminiscence as he limped off the court.

"Hey Andy," one of my pledge brothers said, "play." It was part request, part command.

No way, I thought. Do you guys want to lose? But I thought I might have a little game left in me, and what did it matter? "O.K.," I said.

I slipped out of my jacket and began to play. I was almost instantly exhausted. I kept coughing and wheezing and couldn't catch my breath. I was spitting up chunks of green phlegm. My shirt was soaked in sweat. The game seemed to last for hours. The wind was pushing me around like a rag doll. Finally our team got the ball. It was mine. I shot it. It was an airball. I used to have what some of my fraternity brothers admiringly called "the shot" because it was so accurate. That was gone.

Toward the end of the game, I took breaks at every possession change and was heaving up enough mucus for a whole sick ward. Imagine how much worse it would have been if it was a summer day in Athens where temperatures reach the 100-degree mark regularly. I was minutes from quitting when Brad, one of the fraternity's best players, crouched for a jump shot. I tried to block him. The next thing I felt was a blow that sent me to the ground like a pin in a bowling alley. I didn't know what hit me. I realized I'd been plowed over by a 200-pound muscular player named Brett who was built like a wall. Between coughing spasms, I looked up from the ground to see Brett grinning maliciously.

His beefy hands encircled my skinny bicep and he lifted me off the ground. I had no power to resist him or even to help myself up. I was like a marionette without strings, a limp version of myself.

"Entering any weightlifting contests anytime soon?" Brett said with a sarcastic laugh. Everyone laughed with him. They were laughing at me, as usual. His jab took another cut into what little ego I had left. I was hurt, again. And I was angry. What right did he have to mock me like that?

I shockingly realized that Brett had every right. I was a loser who deserved to be scorned. It wasn't because of CF, though. I was a loser because CF was my excuse for everything that sucked in my life, from my lack of friends and a girlfriend to my bad grades and even worse attitude. By telling myself that I was a failure because of CF, I made myself into one.

I finished that basketball game. It hurt terribly. I gasped for breath with every shot and my throat and chest felt raw from my incessant coughing. My team lost. I was the reason they lost. Everyone headed inside to shower and eat dinner, but I stayed out on the deserted court. The temperature got colder, but I didn't realize how blustery the winds were anymore. I could only reminisce. I remembered other games I'd played there and how my fraternity brothers vied to have me on their team. I remembered when they didn't want to guard me because I was such an accurate shooter. Now, they didn't want to guard me because there was no challenge in it. I was hardly an athlete and even less of a person. I was a sick kid with CF.

What had happened to me in the last eight months? How had I faded from the cool and athletic "Flip" to someone so self-hating and timid, so pitiful and despairing? I'd always had a steady stream of friends calling to invite me out or stopping by to talk. I'd chased them all away and retreated further into myself, seeking their pity. Was I any happier? No. Had I made my peace with CF? Not really. What was I doing? Where was I going?

I turned these thoughts over for so long that the afternoon faded to evening and the lights in the fraternity house and the houses across the street began to pop on. Finally, I pulled myself up from the sofa and slowly walked inside. I wasn't sure what I was going to do.

Inside my room, all the rage I'd been feeling for months welled up inside of me. "Damnit! Damnit! Damnit!" I screamed. "What the hell have I done to myself?" I was so enraged that I ripped off my shirt. "I hate myself! I hate myself!" But then I said something that I hadn't said before or even thought in all those months. I don't know where it came from. It just sort of erupted from within.

"I'm going to change! I mean it! I'm going to change!" The words startled me. How would I change? I looked at myself in the mirror. A pale, nearly gaunt face with red-rimmed eyes and a sad mouth stared back at me. I knew my face so well, yet this seemed like a stranger's. I examined myself as though I was strange. Who was this person? I felt a rush of compassion and an urge to help him. Not pity him, but help him out of the hole he'd fallen into. No more feeling sorry for myself, I vowed, and the face in the mirror nodded solemnly. No more skipping therapy. No more skipping pills. No more skipping meals or classes. No more ...

There was a knock at the door. I opened it and there

was the guy who'd showed me the bag of pot that morning.

"Ready?" he said, grinning.

I was ready, but not for that. It would have been so easy though, to try it just once to escape, even temporarily, from what I knew would be a grueling battle back. I wasn't sure I could do it. Was it even worth attempting? I remembered Brett's sneer and the whispers of "Is he gay?" and the look of horror on the girl's face when she saw me doing my therapy. I remembered the face in the mirror, looking and waiting for – for this?

"Never mind," I told him. "You go ahead, O.K.? I can't risk hurting myself."

His face fell.

"O.K.," he said with a shrug.

This was the first challenge to my new resolve. I'd mastered it. Now, I had to take the next step. I had to make some drastic changes. I grabbed a notebook and a pen and settled down on the sofa. I wanted to make a list: "Ways to improve myself." What did I want? I wanted to play basketball again. And I wanted to play it well. I wanted to have the energy to walk to my classes again. I wanted to attend my classes and bring home a report card I'd be proud to show my parents. I wanted friends and a girlfriend. I looked at my watch. I didn't really notice what time it was because time was irrelevant. The time was now.

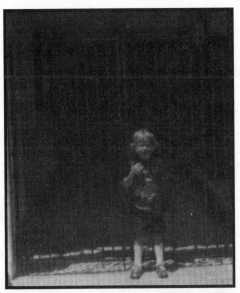

At an early age, Superman was my hero. When the odds were against him, he would still find a way to win. I would soon find out that I would have to have that same relentlessness.

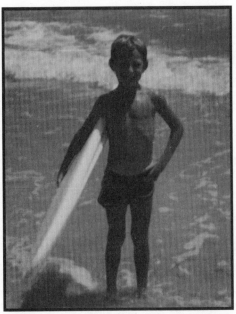

Most children with CF have a tough time gaining weight. As a child, you could see I was having that same difficulty.

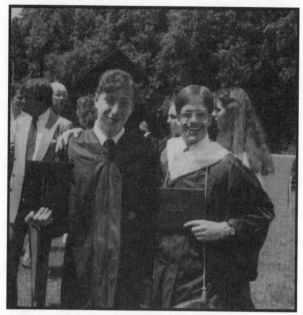

This was Josh and me at our high school graduation in 1991.

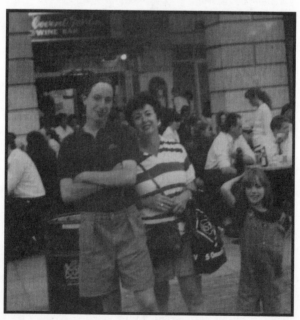

This is a picture of my mom, Emily, and me while we were in Europe.
This was a vacation we took prior to my freshman year at Georgia.

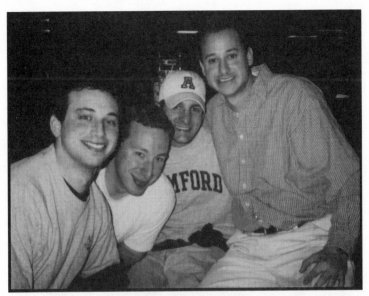

This was a time in which I was battling 3 bacterial infections. But my roommates (from left to right) Peter, Ross, and Wayne got me through a lot of those tough times. In this picture, we had just bowled while a winter stormed knocked out all our power.

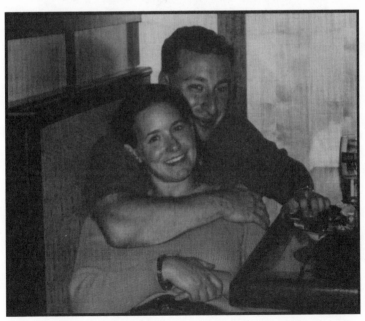

Here is a picture of Andrea and me. We have been together for over a year and she has taught me so much about the person I am and the person I want to be. I love her with all my heart.

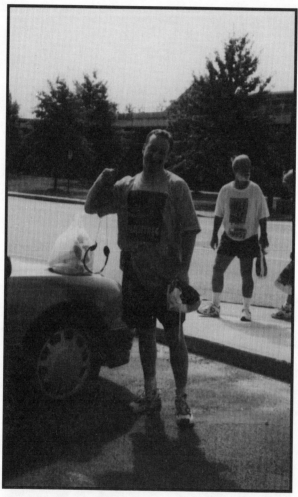

After finishing my 2nd Peachtree, I proudly wore my T-shirt. My Uncle Bobby, who stands behind me with a friend, was behind my Peachtree success.

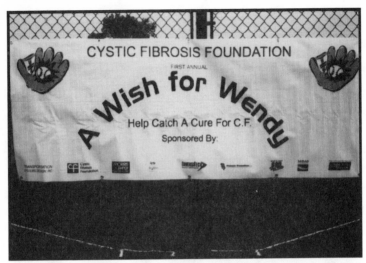

"A Wish for Wendy" raised nearly $40,000 for CF research in its first year of existence. It was the single most important thing I've ever done.

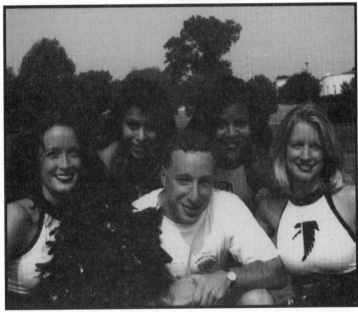

It's tough running a charity event. This is me along with the hired entertainment, the Atlanta Falcon cheerleaders.

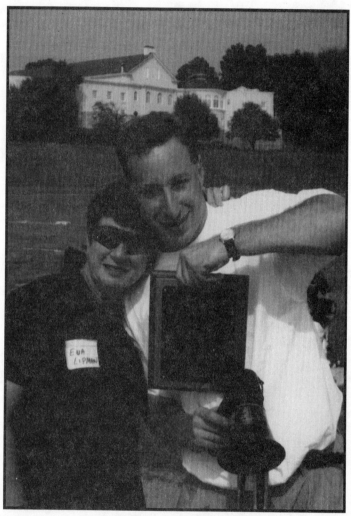

I presented my mom with the "Outstanding Volunteer" award from the CF Foundation last year. But it is small in comparison to the support she gives me every day.

16

LIFTING THE WEIGHT

Winter 1993 – Age 20

When the alarm clock woke me the next morning, something felt different. It took a minute to realize what it was. Today was the day I would begin challenging myself to overcome my doubts, defeat cystic fibrosis, and change the attitude that had been dragging me down.

The most important thing I needed to do that day was register for the next quarter's classes. I signed up for economics and accounting – and advanced weightlifting. I didn't need that class to graduate. I was taking it to help me get through life.

Since entering college, I'd despised my body. I had bony arms and a skinny chest. My legs looked like twigs. I refused to go to go to Legion Pool, the university's swimming area, because I didn't want anyone to see my scrawny frame. I knew the guys would be shedding their shirts and catching rays, so I'd tell my friends I had homework or that my medicine made me too sensitive to the sun. When I played basketball and the teams were split into "shirts" and "skins," I sat that one out. I didn't want girls passing by to see how skinny I was.

On the first day of advanced weightlifting, I nervously entered the gym. I was discouraged to see that I was probably the smallest guy in the class. Most of the guys who'd signed up played on the college football team. Some of them were bigger than my car. I was afraid that if they didn't look where they were going, they might accidentally trample me. I did see with relief, however, that my fraternity brother, Greg, was in the class. He looked as uneasy as I felt, which made me feel better. Everyone chatted as they waited for class to start when suddenly someone bellowed, "Everyone quiet!"

Coach Miller* entered the room. He was only 5-foot-6, but had forearms that looked like they could bend lead. "Everyone, sit down and shut up!" he hollered. I figured that this would be much like prison or boot camp.

"I have three rules in my class," the coach said, eyeing us as though we were serving life sentences for murder. "First of all, no excuses if you're late. If you are tardy, you'll do a mile's worth of laps around the track. If you're late again, I'll double it. If you're late again, you'll fail."

"Second rule: You have to be here for every class. If you miss a day, you have to run the track. If you miss another day, you'll run farther. Miss three days—"

I knew where this was going.

"—and you fail. My third rule is that everyone must participate. One person will count each day as we do pushups. If you lose count, the rest of the class will start over. If you can't finish, you'll start over. Is this clear?"

"Yes sir," we chimed in unison. My mouth said yes, but my brain was objecting. What was I getting myself into?

Next, Coach Miller handed out disclaimer forms which asked us to list any health problems or illnesses. Not long ago, I would have written "I have cystic fibrosis" on the form. Today, I wrote "none." I'd have no excuse for not excelling.

Coach Miller then said he'd group us based on how much weight we could lift. Greg lifted about 175 pounds. I had a hunch I wouldn't be in his group. I'd never lifted weights in high school, unless you counted my algebra book. I did know how to lift a 45-pound barbell from watching Josh when we were freshmen.

While Coach Miller watched, I lifted 45 pounds. Then 65, 85, and 105 pounds. I couldn't quite lift 115, but felt good with what I was able to lift. Then I saw that some of the girls in the class could lift that much as well. I wondered if I was making a mistake by continuing the course.

Coach Miller told me that by the time the 10-week

class ended, he'd like me to be able to lift 155 pounds.
I decided I'd reach for 165. It was the first time in a
while that my expectations exceeded someone else's
concerning my abilities.

That afternoon I went to a sporting goods store and
bought workout gloves, Spandex shorts, and some T-
shirts. I wanted to look the part of a weightlifter for an
extra boost of confidence. Those gloves got some use. I
lifted weights every day of class, like we were supposed
to do. I did pull-ups, push-ups, dips, curls, and everything else Coach Miller ordered. He always demanded
more, and I realized I thrived on that challenge. Some
days I'd crawl out of class feeling like a jellyfish – wob-
bly and limp. But I didn't quit. Sometimes I even went
to the gym on weekends. If Coach Mervos said to do 10
sets, I'd do 11. If he called for 12 repetitions, I did 13.
For the first time in so long, I was driven to succeed.

I would love to say that everything went smoothly,
that I bulked up and everyone was inspired by me. Of
course, it wasn't quite that easy. One afternoon, a
bunch of us were watching a baseball game on TV at
the fraternity. Brian, a die-hard weightlifter, glanced
over at me and grimaced.

"Andy," he said, "you really shouldn't roll up your
sleeves like that until you get some muscles."

Everyone looked at my arms, and I knew they were
thinking what I was thinking: scrawny. The guys
chuckled. A few weeks ago, I would have stormed out
of the room. This time, though my pride was wound-

ed, I simply bit my lip and kept my mouth shut. Brian's comment made me realize I'd have to keep working to see results. After he teased me, I never rolled up my sleeves. Later on, when someone told me with admiration that I was bulking up, I'd shrug and say that my shirt was tight.

The second goal I set during weightlifting was to walk to class without sounding and feeling like I had emphysema. I didn't share this goal with anyone because I didn't want them to know I felt exhausted after walking even a quarter of a mile. I had often bummed rides from my fraternity brothers, saying I hurt my leg or I had to be in class early. I didn't want to admit how weak I was. I had even looked into taking what was called the "disability bus." The woman at the clinic told me it stopped right by the fraternity house. It seemed like a good idea – until I saw that girl.

I watched the bus pull into the nearby parking lot. A girl in a wheelchair got on using her mouth to guide her chair's controls. She did not even look up because she had to concentrate on maneuvering her wheelchair onto the bus. She may have appeared disabled, but she was emotionally stronger than I was. She was getting where she had to go. My handicap was nonexistent compared to hers. Mine was all mental. I'd call it an Andy-cap. After seeing how courageously she handled herself, I realized I couldn't ask for a ride on the bus. I was simply looking for an excuse, and in the process, appropriating a service that should be available for people who didn't have other options. I didn't need a bus to take me to class.

The only way to get to class on time was to leave at least 15 minutes early. That way I could take breaks to catch my breath, cough, or spit up phlegm. Every day I walked, and every day I coughed and huffed and puffed. Friends saw me and offered rides, but I always declined. They may have thought I was being rude. Maybe I should have explained my goal, but I was so unsure of whether it was attainable that I didn't want to tell anyone for fear I'd fail and they'd remember.

By the end of the quarter, I could walk to class without gasping. I realized I looked better from all the weight-lifting and training and I felt better too. I was doing my therapy daily and taking all my necessary medicines. I began eating better. Not that I couldn't have lived on Shoney's strawberry pies. But I knew that if I was going to get strong and stay that way, I needed to put high-test fuel in the engine. The better I felt, the happier I was.

At our last weight-lifting class, it was time to examine our progress. There was only one way to measure our success —compare how much weight we could lift in our last class to the weight we had lifted in our first class. I knew I looked better, but I remembered Brian's remark and worried that maybe I hadn't improved as much as I had thought. That day, I lifted weights of different sizes, including 155 pounds, the goal Coach Miller had set for me. I brought the weight to my chest and heaved it back onto the bar. I was sweating, but I'd done it. I'd reached that goal. Now I needed another. I asked for another 15 pounds on the bar.

"Are you sure?" asked the guy who was spotting me. I looked exhausted. I was panting from the exertion of lifting, and my forehead and chest were damp with sweat. But my spirit was rejuvenated.

"Yup," I said, "put it on there."

I settled myself on the bench, took a few deep breaths, and closed my eyes to gather my energy. I slowly counted to three and then lifted. I lowered the bar to my chest and put everything I had into lifting it. I thought about Brett and about people who doubted me. As I lifted the weight, I pushed them and their negativity up and away. For all that was balanced on the bar, it was surprisingly light. And I'd exceeded my personal goal by lifting 170 pounds.

At the end of class, Coach Miller went around the room and asked everyone to state our starting weight, then the weight he had expected us to lift in the final class, and then the weight we had actually lifted. When he said "Andy Lipman," I replied proudly, "105 pounds, 155 pounds, and 170 pounds." My fraternity brother Greg gave me a respectful smile. That was something I hadn't seen in a long, long time.

I felt so happy I practically skipped home. I called Aunt Susie that night to tell her about the 170 pounds. "I'm back," I said with a laugh. "I'm back."

My health had improved. I was taking my medication and doing my therapy. I was on the antibiotics that my doctor prescribed. After several weeks of hard work, my phlegm was clear again and I returned to sleeping on my loft. My grades improved that quarter along with my attendance. Hmmm. I'm sure they were related. I understood more of the lectures, and my classes became more interesting. I began spending time in a place I hadn't seen much since my freshman year. It was called the library. I fell into a routine that I enjoyed. Classes in the morning. Gym in the afternoon. Library at night.

My fraternity brothers noticed these changes. I stopped feeling sorry for myself. I didn't expect anyone else to feel sorry for me either. I wanted friendship and company. I wanted to be treated like one of them, and that meant not pitying or distancing myself. I stopped hiding out in my room, and when someone was brave enough to ask "the recluse" if he wanted to go out for a bite or catch a movie, I swallowed my fears that they were asking only because they pitied me – and said O.K. The more I said yes, the less hesitancy I had about making friends and the more likely they were to invite me again. I tried to make a special effort with Josh. I had basically thrown his friendship away during my depression and he had noticed. In fact, he had called my mom several times fearing that my life was in danger. Now, however, we were back on track. We started to spend many days together at the gym and the library.

I was elected vice president of TEP and became the fraternity's athletic chairman and pledge trainer. The biggest surprise was that during my senior year, I was named "most congenial brother," despite some of those bitter confrontations during my sophomore and junior years. That meant a lot to me. It made me realize that my newfound strengths weren't unnoticed by those who saw me every day and knew me best. I was making more time for my friends and having more intimate conversations with them. As a result, they saw me as a person who they wanted to represent them. But there was still one score to settle.

17

REVENGE

Spring 2004 – Age 20

To the other five guys who played basketball at TEP that day, it was simply another game being played – a way to get some exercise, blow off some steam, and hang out. To me, though, it was literally a shot at redemption.

I hadn't planned to play that afternoon. What I really wanted was a shower and a tall glass of ice water. I'd been working out at the gym and I was exhausted. I flopped down on the sofa by the basketball court, content to sun myself and watch my fraternity brothers vie for baskets.

I didn't expect them to ask me to play. I couldn't forget the humiliation I had felt several months ago when Brett plowed me over and then mockingly scraped me up off the asphalt like curbside litter. I wondered if they remembered that day as keenly as I did.

But you can't play three-on-three with just five guys.
So when one guy gasped that he'd had enough and
headed inside, everyone on the court looked to me. In
those few months, I'd developed some pride and a much
stronger upper body. I was willing to play, not only to
prove that I could, but also because I had a score to settle. This was my chance to set the record straight. One
of the players on the other team was Brett. My opponents that day were Brett and cystic fibrosis.

Despite my gym workout before the game, I felt
energized and lively as soon as the game began. I was
alert and quick, grabbing the ball and shooting.
Sometimes I nailed the basket and sometimes I missed,
but I never felt wheezy. I moved with the confidence
and vigor I'd been lacking since the last time I set foot
on the court.

The game was in its final minutes when Brett got
the ball.

"Shoot it!" someone yelled.

He never got the chance. As he aimed the ball, a 5-
foot-8 150-pound kid on my team slammed into him.
His feet flew out from under him and he fell onto the
unforgiving asphalt. He looked stunned, especially as
my teammate sank a jump shot with the same ball he'd
been holding only seconds before. The 150 pound kid
– that was me!

"Take that," I thought, glaring down at him. "No
one's ever knocking me down again."

Brett raised his hand to me, implying that he wanted me to pull him up, but I ignored the unspoken request.

"Get your own self up," I muttered as I walked away and wiped my hands on my shorts. For the first time in a long time, I was standing up for myself.

I don't remember who won the game. It doesn't really matter, does it? I won because I showed that I wouldn't let cystic fibrosis or anyone get the best of me. When we finished, we all gave each other high gives, a TEP tradition. Brett and I slapped our sweaty palms together, and he mentioned that I looked like I'd been working out because my chest had broadened. I knew that was his way of apologizing. I found myself feeling a bit of appreciation for his motivation. His disparaging comments ultimately turned me around.

I ambled up to my room so that no one would think the basketball game was a big deal. But as soon as I shut the door, I cranked up "Eye of the Tiger," ripped off my T-shirt, and danced like Michael Jackson. "I did it," I told myself. "I showed him. I showed them all."

I caught a glimpse of myself in the mirror and, for the first time in a long time, was pleased with what I saw. Grinning back at me was a slightly red-faced, slightly breathless guy with strong arms and a muscular chest, and he was radiating an unmistakable confidence.

18

OH, DIOS

Summer 1995 – Age 21

I shared an apartment in Athens my senior year with Haim, a fraternity brother from Miami. He was a great roommate, maybe the best I ever had. We both loved sports, food, and exercise and got along like brothers – or how I assumed brothers would get along. Not having one, I couldn't really say, but anyone who was as close to his brother as Haim and I were was a lucky guy.

I never thought Haim would witness one of the most frightening experiences of my life. Fortunately for me, he wasn't just a bystander, but someone who took charge of the situation. Who knows what would have happened if he hadn't?

Haim was the quarterback of our pledge football team and I was one of the wide receivers. He used to tease me that the only good thing about my hands was that I never dropped the cup of water I handed him on the sidelines. I used to tell him that the great thing about him was that he was free of prejudice; he threw the ball to both our teammates and our opponents.

What Haim lacked on the gridiron, he made up for in the kitchen. This guy could cook. He made dinner almost every night and I did the dishes. It was like living with my mom, but without any interrogations. Haim's cooking skills didn't rub off on me, but his diligence certainly did. The summer of 1995, before our fifth year, he studied at least four hours every night for the medical school admission test. He was already taking classes during the day and working out regularly. Plus, like me, he was in a long-distance relationship. His girlfriend was interning in Atlanta for the summer.

Bryna, my first serious girlfriend, was studying in Europe that summer. And Josh had graduated, so I was really feeling lonely. Haim more than made up for their absence. We talked about the difficulties of long-distance relationships, and we debated endlessly about who was a better athlete. We lifted weights together at least once a week. And we ate like food was an endangered species.

My family liked Haim, too. Whenever my dad came to visit, he took Haim and I to the grocery store and loaded about 20 frozen meals into the cart. I'd tell my dad we had enough, but Haim would give me a look that would shut me up, and he'd drop in another armful or two. Haim was notorious around our fraternity house as a world-class eater. Of course, I was no slouch either.

That summer, we planned a July Fourth barbecue. Of course, Haim was going to man the grill. I couldn't wait. He made the most amazing ribs and chicken. I was ready for a feast. I popped three Pancrease pills, an enzyme to help CFers digest the fat in food. The more you plan to eat, the more you should take because otherwise you can't physiologically break down fat. I've been taking these pills for as long as I can remember, since my mom put them in applesauce so I could swallow them.

This time, though, I seriously underestimated how much I'd eat. I devoured 10 ribs, four pieces of chicken, some rice, and some corn. The food smelled so good and it just kept coming, and we were all kicking back, reminiscing about our years in college and speculating about where we'd be in 10 years. I didn't think about what I was eating.

I woke up the next morning with a mild stomach ache. I sat on the toilet for a half an hour, but to no avail. Constipated. Damn. I went to class anyway. Summer school was starting, and I wanted to make a good impression. As the day progressed, however, the pain worsened. Just sitting in class was painful. I remembered that throbbing hurt all too well. One time in grade school, my mom had to give me enemas for an entire week. No way I was going through that again.

After my last class, I went straight to the student health center. You can guess how desperate I was. The joke around campus was that whether you were suffering from a heart attack or a sore throat, you'd get the same treatment: a prescription for amoxicillin and instructions to take it easy.

I told the doctor my problem and that I had CF. I could see in his eyes that he was unnerved. I imagined him thinking: "CF! Hmm... Now what did we learn in medical school about CF? Aha! Where's that amoxicillin?" He told me I ate too much – well, I knew that! – and told me to lie on my side. He pulled a plastic glove onto his hand and then stuck his hand into my rectum and removed the feces stuck inside me. Then he gave me a barium enema to clean out what remained.

It sounds gross, and it was. When he was done, I couldn't look him in the eye, but I felt so much better. There was just a slight pain in my stomach, but the doctor said it was normal. I swore to myself that no matter how tantalizing the food looked at a barbecue, restaurant, or my parents' house, I'd never, ever eat like that again.

When I got home, I told Haim about my big adventure, though I spared him some of the details. I felt so much better that I worked out and then studied. It was a tough and embarrassing day, but I still felt good because I'd taken care of myself and my health on my own. My mom tends to be overprotective, but this experience proved to me that I was capable of watching out for my own health. I was proud of myself.

All that changed the next morning. I woke up in even more pain than the day before. I struggled through my morning classes and that afternoon, I went back to the health center. The doctor who I'd seen the day before wasn't there, but a nurse gave me several barium enemas. She asked me if the pain stopped. I told her it had, but I was lying. Honestly, I just wanted to get the hell out of there. Being naked – intensely naked, you might say – in front of a nurse might appear on somebody's radar as a bizarre fantasy, but for me, it was pure horror. I'd had enough.

I staggered home and fell into bed. I couldn't sleep and I didn't know how to ease the pain. I didn't want to go through the whole humiliating experience again at a hospital, and I definitely did not want to call my folks. I was an adult and I could take care of myself. Right?

When Haim got home he knew something was wrong, though I insisted I was fine. He made Chinese food and brought it up to my room, but I couldn't eat more than a few bites. When he saw that I wasn't eating, he looked at me warily. "I ate earlier," I lied.

My parents called about a half an hour later to say goodbye before their trip to Israel the next day. My mom suspected something was wrong. But I didn't want her to know how terrible I felt because then they'd panic, rush to see me, and cancel their trip. I assured her I was fine, and she seemed persuaded. But after we hung up the phone, I thought about my situation. What if I didn't feel any better the next day? My folks would be overseas. My doctor, who no longer worked at the University of North Carolina, was in Cincinnati. What the heck would I do?

When the phone rang again, Haim grabbed it. "Andy has a terrible stomach ache," I heard him say. "Since Monday." My mom must've asked him if he thought they should come because my buddy, the guy who was studying to get into podiatry school – and did – said, "It's probably a good idea."

My parents arrived several hours later, and I realized just how desperately I needed their help. Luckily for me, they're veterans when it comes to dealing with my medical emergencies. Paramedics have nothing on my folks. They immediately called Dr. Boat and told him what was going on. He said I needed to drink a jug of a liquid called Golytely, the stuff a stomach surgery patient drinks before his or her operation.

At that point, I was all for it. Bring on the medical cocktail. I'd already had more enemas than I could count, some courtesy of a female nurse. This couldn't be any worse, right? I wouldn't even have to get undressed. Turns out Golytely is the worst-tasting stuff I've ever swallowed. It could be used for enemy torture. It was clear, but viscous like mineral oil and tasted like the week-old milk I once accidentally drank in high school. I managed to choke down five glasses before I started crying.

"I can't drink any more," I sobbed. "This stuff sucks. I'm going to throw up."

My mom looked just as upset as I felt, but she knew the situation was serious. "Drink it," she urged, "or we'll have to take you to the hospital." "O.K.," I sobbed. I think that was the only time ever I didn't offer a word of objection when my folks wanted to take me to a doctor. I couldn't stop crying. I was doubled over in pain. My parents, one on each side, practically carried me to the car. I remember seeing the look of terror on Haim's face as my parents guided me out.

At St. Mary's Hospital, my mom maneuvered me into a wheelchair and we waited in the emergency room. I begged each nurse who passed by to help me. I screamed, "Help me! Please! Help me! Please! Why won't they help me? Why? It hurts! It hurts!" I felt like a homeless man begging for change from passersby who continued to ignore him.

After what seemed like an eternity, a nurse called my name. I was wheeled into a room where a doctor asked me a long list of questions. He hooked me up to an IV to ease my pain and prepare me for the operating room. I don't remember much, thank goodness, but I do remember the bright lights and the sensation of having my pants unzipped and pulled off my legs. Here we go again with the enemas. At least I didn't have to look anyone in the eye. Eventually, I was cleaned out. Exhausted, I was sent home with orders to always match my enzyme intake to my food intake. It was definitely a lesson that stuck.

My condition, I learned years later from a CF medical book, was called distal intestinal obstruction syndrome, or DIOS. It's fairly common among people with CF, and it's tied to not taking enough enzymes with meals. I remember from Spanish class that "Dios" means God. My experience was pretty ungodly, I'd say.

I spent five days in Atlanta with my folks, recuperating slowly. Fortunately, my pain was gone. But so was my energy. I felt wiped out, physically and emotionally. My dad drove me back to school and urged me to take it easy. Then he and my mom went on their trip to Israel. Haim said he was glad to see me and told me I needed to go to the gym to get my strength back.

I shook my head in frustration. "I can't," I told him, recounting the long tale of the enemas, the pain, and the humiliation.

"C'mon, man. Don't be lazy," he said.

That was all I needed to hear. Me, lazy? Not a chance.

I hauled my weary butt out of bed. I worked out that day for the first time in at least a week, and I worked out the rest of the week too. I got back into the groove of studying, spending three or four hours a night on my classes. It shouldn't be any big surprise that my grades picked up. In fact, I made all As that quarter. Haim's impressive study habits rubbed off on me. So did his dedication to fitness. By the end of the summer, I was in the best shape I'd ever been in.

As fall rolled around and the rest of the students arrived on campus, I realized I'd had a heck of a summer. I'd fought DIOS in one of the toughest CF battles I'd had since the meconium ileus at my birth (and I can't take credit for that because I don't remember it), and I realized that whatever punches CF threw at me, I could face them, duck them, and dodge them. I'd stared down my opponent, and though it got a few good hits in at me, I was still standing. And I looked pretty darn good in the ring.

You might say that July 4, 1995, was an Independence Day for me, too. CF didn't control my life, and I could beat it if I put my mind to it. I had plans for the next July 4, too – a little something to keep CF on the run, you might say.

19

THE T-SHIRT

Summer 1985 – Age 11

Every time my Uncle Bobby wore his Peachtree Road Race T-shirt, I swear my mouth watered. People saw him wearing it and asked all kinds of questions: "Bobby, how long did you train?" "What was your time?" "How many races have you run in?" He'd always have a story about the smothering heat on race day or his fellow runners or the exhaustion he faced as he neared the finish line. I wished I could be the one telling those stories.

The Peachtree, as it's called, is the biggest 10K race in the world. It brings tens of thousands of runners to the city each July 4th. Police close off the 6.2 miles of road and runners take over. Thousands of cheering fans line the streets with signs and cups of water for the runners. Many are professionals from around the world who whip across the finish line with astounding times.

Most, however, are people you'd see running in the neighborhood, joggers and runners who set their sights on a goal and move toward it.

Everyone who crosses the finish line at Piedmont Park, the big downtown park, receives a Peachtree Road Race T-shirt. You can't buy them, and no runner who's finished the race would ever give theirs away. The only way to get one is to run the race.

Bobby had about 18 Peachtree T-shirts, which really was no surprise. He had been a football coach at Georgia State and had run in the Boston and New York marathons. He was very big on motivation. If you weren't motivated, you didn't earn his respect. Though he was married to my Aunt Susie, I never really liked Bobby much because he was so tough on me.

Other relatives, knowing I had CF, might want to coddle me, but Bobby would have none of that. My father and I would play my aunt and uncle in doubles, and they'd always win. The two of them combined had more trophies than I had excuses. I was so envious of the easy grace he seemed to have on every court, be it tennis or basketball. He didn't have to work as hard as I did, it seemed, and yet he continued to whip my butt.

It really irked me that I couldn't beat him in tennis, and he certainly wasn't going to throw a game my way out of sympathy. With Bobby, if you were going to win, you had to earn it. That made me resent him, but it also, grudgingly, strengthened my lasting respect for him. More than ever, I wanted to beat him, because in some way, I figured, that would be like beating CF.

True to his nature as a coach, Bobby was glad to help me shape up athletically, though he often did it with sarcasm. He'd build up a big lead on me and then launch into "Your mama's so fat ..." jokes just to deepen the insult. But, hey, it worked. Bobby helped me train nearly every day when I was a student at Mt. Vernon Presbyterian School. As a result of his dedication, I went from finishing last in my class in running laps from the first to the fourth grade to finishing among the top three runners in fifth grade. For the first time in my life, I was one of the first kids chosen when teams were picked. I looked forward to gym and recess. I was even named "most improved athlete" when I was 10.

Yet it wasn't enough. I still couldn't beat him. So I decided to join him. I wanted to earn a Peachtree T-shirt, and I knew that, despite the taunts, Bobby would be the best person to train and motivate me.

We began when I was 11 with two or three miles at a time, twice a week. It took nearly six months to build up to five miles, almost the length of the race itself, which includes, of course, Peachtree Road, Atlanta's most famous street. And I did it. I went to sleep thinking about how good it would feel to wear the race T-shirt that I'd earn in less than two weeks.

The next day, I ran another five miles and then played tennis with Josh for an hour and a half. When I stretched to hit a ball, I felt a weird twinge in my right ankle. It didn't really hurt so I kept playing, but later

that night it still felt strange. The next morning, I could-
n't walk without limping. Instead of going away, the
pain only worsened. I refused to see a doctor and decided I'd sit this one out. I think I was more scared than
hurt, honestly. I reluctantly told Bobby he'd have to
train without me. He was disappointed because he
never doubted I had the ability to run the race. He did-
n't want me to give up, but he also knew that I had to
have confidence in my own abilities.

As each day passed, my confidence eroded a little
more. It was gone when, about a week before the race,
I lost my number, my ticket to the Peachtree. My parents sold it out from under me to a runner who hadn't
gotten one of the coveted numbers. Because the race is
so popular, there aren't enough spaces for everyone
who wants to run. Since the demand for numbers is so
high, people can and do actually buy numbers from
people who aren't running.

As soon as this woman merrily handed her $12 to
my parents, I realized my dream of running that year's
Peachtree was really, truly gone. She smiled at me,
grateful for a ticket to the race. But I glared back. "You
should be ashamed," I thought, "for taking a kid's
number. You took my T-shirt. You took my dream."
Deep inside, though, I knew this runner was nothing
more than a bystander in the internal battle I was constantly fighting with myself.

On the morning of July 4th, I watched the race on
TV. I couldn't bear to join the crowds downtown urg-

ing the runners on. The cameras were fixed on the finish line, where runner after runner joyously pumped their arms into the air with expressions of victory and the accomplishment. I sobbed.

Bobby called me that afternoon. "Have a good sleep?" he teased, knowing that if I'd been running the race, I would have been up before 6 a.m.

"Just fine," I said. "I don't care about some stupid race. I'll run it next year."

But I didn't. Or the year after. Or after that, either. Instead, I concentrated on tennis. When I was 14, I even did the previously impossible: I defeated my mortal enemy, Uncle Bobby, after hundreds of losses. With every point I won, I felt a changing of the guard. After all these years, I was the athlete in the family. Well, not quite. Bobby still had a whole drawer of Peachtree Road Race T-shirts. I had a drawer full of polo shirts. And Bobby was just the type of person to remind me of that.

In 1996, when I was nearly 22, I decided it was time. I called Bobby and told him: "I'm going to put on that T-shirt."

He knew exactly what I was talking about.

"We'll see," he said. "You've said that before. Why should this time be any different?"

I paused.

"Because I want it. I really want it. See you on the Fourth."

Aunt Susie got on the phone.

"Andy, honey," she said. "You know you don't have

to run the whole thing, or any of it. You can walk and get that T-shirt. That's O.K. too."

"If I'm going to enter the Peachtree, I'm going to run it," I said, annoyed that she was so quick to cut her nephew a break. "I don't do things half-assed."

When the race applications appeared in the Atlanta newspaper, I immediately filled one out and mailed it in. I could picture myself crossing the finish line and my uncle picking me up on his shoulders and parading me around. Friends would be cheering at my victory, and I might be sweaty and tired, but I'd wear my new T-shirt, the one I earned with every step, to breakfast that morning.

It was a good fantasy. I had a ways to go to make it a reality. I hadn't even started to train for the race. I figured that when I got my number, that would be the green light I needed to start working toward my goal.

An envelope from the race officials arrived a month later. I decided to hang the race number it contained on my bulletin board to motivate me. But there was no race number inside. Instead, there was a form letter. My application had been rejected because I forgot to send a picture I.D. I was dumbfounded.

I should have blamed myself for not reading the application carefully enough. Instead, I vented all my rage on my mom. "Why didn't you tell me I needed to send a picture I.D.?" I demanded.

"Andy, I can't do everything. You filled out the application. You should have read it more carefully.

Why don't you call them and see if you can..."

"Forget it," I sulked. "I'll just skip it again. It's only a stupid race."

That July 4th, Bobby was in his usual fine form. "Did you see me on TV?" he gloated. "How did I look? I'm glad you almost ran it again this year."

After I hung up the phone, I thought of what I should have said: "I almost run it every year."

20

THE BOOKMARK

Summer 1996 – Age 22

Nearly a year later, I'd graduated from the University of Georgia and returned to Atlanta. I still had boxes of stuff from my college apartment. I figured my baseball cards, all 50,000 of them, must be in there somewhere, so on a Saturday when there was nothing on TV, I began digging through the boxes. Something I found amid the Nerf basketball net and baseball caps restored my drive to run the Peachtree.

It was a bookmark shaped like a tennis racket. I'd forgotten I saved it, but I remembered exactly when I received it. I was 17 and was helping out with the bartending at my dad's company party. Becky Decker, his secretary, wished me a happy birthday and told me she heard I'd made the school's tennis team. The bookmark, she said, would remind me to do my best at school and tennis. I didn't know Becky well, but I knew enough from my dad to know that Becky was one of the most thoughtful people around. The fact she not only remembered my birthday, but remembered my interests said a lot about her.

A few years later when I was in college, my mother sadly told me that Becky had cancer. How could that be? I was the one with the incurable disease, and she was an effervescent person who lit up any room she entered. She died a few months later. My dad gave the eulogy at her funeral and framed a poem he had written about her and hung it in the office conference room.

I remembered Becky's words when she gave me the bookmark: "...do your best..." Had I really done my best? Not when it came to the Peachtree Road Race. I dialed Bobby's number, my speed increasing with each digit I punched, before I could change my mind.

He chuckled. "You're kidding, right?" Same old Bobby.

"Let's pretend I'm not," I said. "I want your help."

"O.K.," he said. "Start with running once a week. Run for time, not distance. Build your stamina. Don't worry how far or how fast. Just go. And run on the street. Don't use a treadmill; it won't help you learn how to handle hills." Bobby offered to run with me, but I wanted to run alone. I wanted to train at my pace. This was my Peachtree.

I began training in January 1997, a good six months before race day. On a chilly Saturday morning, I walked outside, stretched, and set off on a slow jog. God, it felt good to be running again. My feet hit the street rhythmically and the air was crisp and fresh.

Who was I kidding? A quarter-mile from home, I was slammed by a severe coughing attack. I doubled over, spitting thick gobs of phlegm onto the street. When the attack subsided, I could barely breathe. I couldn't run anymore. I stopped and limped a few feet toward home. Wrenched by another coughing fit, I heaved up more phlegm. I was soaked in sweat. I sat on the side of the street and then, slowly, made my way home. Damn cystic fibrosis!

I began training every other day. When I could run a quarter-mile, I pushed the distance to a half-mile. Then, a mile. I was one-sixth of the way there. I was still coughing out of control sometimes, but each time I called Bobby to update him on my progress, a little more confidence spread through me. "You're on your way," he said at the end of one of our chats. That's as close as Bobby gets to praise, and hearing it, I thought maybe he believed in me too. A few weeks later, I knew he believed in me. He'd purchased me a membership in the Atlanta Track Club, a club whose members have an edge in being chosen for the race because their entry forms are sent to them before applications became available to everyone in the newspaper.

A week later, when the application for the race appeared in the paper, I filled it out immediately and wrote my $18 check. This time, I remembered to include a picture I.D. After my last devastating experience, there's no way I would have forgotten that! Then I examined a dozen mailboxes in my neighborhood to see which had the earliest mail pickup, because the postmark date can be critical in getting a number for the race.

Before I dropped the envelope down the mail chute, I prayed right there on the sidewalk: "Please, God, let my application go through. I've never wanted anything more than to run in this race. I want Bobby's respect. I want to do this for Becky. Please." Somebody heard my prayer.

By spring, I was up to two-and-a-half miles as often as three times a week. Then, in late May, I did something stupid. Though Bobby had told me not to run on the treadmill, one night I was watching a movie while jogging barefoot on the treadmill. I was surprised to see I'd covered more than four miles. Just two more would be the distance of the Peachtree. Could I do it? I've never met a challenge I didn't like. I stopped when I hit seven miles.

The next morning was payback time for jogging barefoot. What a moron! I couldn't bend my knees. At work, I could barely hobble. I had to sit down and rest with every few steps. I had to wear a brace on each knee when I played outfield on my softball team. I even had to take myself out of a game because the pain was so intense. I'd ice my knees every night and wake up each morning in more pain.

Of course, I didn't go to a doctor, though it would have been a wise idea. I'd like to say I've got nothing against doctors, but after spending so much time with them when I was a child, these days I honestly prefer to let them get some time in with other patients.

I'm sure a doctor would have warned me to take a breather from running for a few weeks. But I knew if I gave up now, I'd never be ready for the race I had my heart set on. And honestly, I couldn't handle another "I told you so" from Bobby. Two weeks after my knee pain, despite the injury, I forced myself to run again. And I felt O.K. Finally over the "Peachtree Hex," I told myself proudly. I wiped the sweat from my face with my hand, and my hand was smeared with red. My nose was gushing blood so badly that I had to peel off my T-shirt and use it to stop the bleeding. My knees were swollen. Was this God's way of telling me to just give up on the race? The wrenched ankle. The application problem. Now this.

Full of self-pity, I called my girlfriend Stephanie to commiserate. Actually, I was supposed to call her earlier, but I was so preoccupied with the race that I'd forgotten. She was furious. She was on vacation and she'd canceled her plans just to talk to me, and I'd never called. Our argument escalated, and we broke up over the phone. I slammed down the receiver and cried.

So three weeks later, what was I doing on Bobby's doorstep on the night of July 3rd, my gym bag in one hand and my running shoes in the other? I wasn't sure I could finish the Peachtree. All I knew was I had to at least start. I thought of Becky, the bookmark, and her urging me to do my best.

After a massive spaghetti dinner, Bobby and I were asleep by 10 p.m. My alarm was set for 4:30 a.m., but I couldn't sleep. I must have, though, because Aunt Susie woke me up by rubbing my shoulder and saying, "Today's the day!"

The sky was still dark at 6:30 a.m. when we arrived at the starting area. The moon was out and the crickets were yielding to the first birds of the morning. I turned on my walkman for some of the tunes on my mixed tape to get me pumped: "Eye of the Tiger," "Jump," and "Welcome to the Jungle." I adjusted my knee braces – in black and red, University of Georgia colors – and wrapped Becky's bookmark around my wrist, tucking it under my wristband. "I admire you, Becky," I thought to her, "and my effort is in your honor."

Before I even crossed the starting line, I was sweating and my knees were sore. Bobby was trying to be supportive, but every time he said, "Relax, big boy. You're gonna be fine," I got more stressed. So much was riding on me: the desire to prove myself to me and to my family and the memories of Becky and her fight against cancer.

I drew energy from the crowd. People were clapping and singing. Some held up signs with the names of family members and friends in the race. One man was wearing a shirt that said, "I had a heart attack one year ago, and here I am today." Everyone who passed him patted him on the back in support. Seeing the cheering spectators, Bobby suggested, "Let the crowd take you to the finish line."

So off we went. I felt great at the one-mile mark. One-sixth of the way there. Knees fine, adrenaline good. Two mile mark: a third of the way there. A few coughs, but nothing serious.

At the two-and-a-half mile mark, I saw signs saying, "Go Bobby and Andy!" My parents, Aunt Susie, cousins Erin and Drew and even Stephanie were there cheering. Though there was no question that Stephanie and I had broken up, there she was. She knew how important that T-shirt was to me, and she hadn't forgotten. My folks took pictures as Bobby and I ran by.

Four miles: Heartbreak Hill, the toughest part of the race. It's a half-mile up, and it's where many of the 20,000 runners walk or even quit. There were a couple times in the past few years when runners had heart attacks there or even died. But I kept running. This race had become a one-on-one fight against cystic fibrosis. I felt a little winded, but I didn't dare stop. I coughed up some phlegm. I kept going. If CF couldn't stop me, Heartbreak Hill certainly couldn't.

Five miles: The end was in sight. I began waving my fist and clapping along with the crowd. With each step, I was closer to the finish line. I was on the verge of finishing a 10K run, more than a 10K, the Peachtree. And I couldn't even walk to class several years ago.

Six miles: My knees began to swell and the pain was intense. We entered Piedmont Park, and I had just a fifth of a mile to go. God, it hurt. Instead of slowing down or even walking, I did something Bobby warned me never to do. I sprinted to the finish line. I took off like a racecar in pursuit of the checkered flag. I did it!

Like everyone else who completed the race, I received a 1997 Peachtree Road Race T-shirt. Bobby, who finished a few seconds behind me, added another T-shirt to his collection.

"Congratulations, big man," he said, sweaty and breathless, but smiling. "I'm proud of you. I told you that you could do it." I'd finally earned his respect by following through on a promise I made nearly a decade before.

We picked our way through the sweaty crowd of runners and supporters. It was nearly noon. My parents were both in tears. I hugged them both, which was out of character, but absolutely right.

I should explain that I never hug my dad. Since my first Little League tryout, we have this sort of under-standing that a handshake is as good as a hug. It was that way, too, with my dad and his dad. On this day, however, we gripped each other and just held tight.

On the way home for much-needed showers, Bobby asked me, "Are you satisfied now that you have your T-shirt?" But satisfaction seems to elude me. As soon as I accomplish something, I set a new goal. There's a sign in my office that says, "Success is a journey, not a destination." It keeps me striving, though sometimes I realize I don't take enough time to enjoy the victories along the way, like finishing a race I'd always dreamed of running.

There would have been nothing shameful about answering Bobby with "Yeah, I'm satisfied – for now." Instead, almost to spite myself, I raised the bar even higher. I told myself that I wouldn't wear this shirt until I ran my next Peachtree and earned another.

21

DATING: IT'S AN ATTITUDE

Fall 1994 – Age 21

I first saw Bryna on the Tau Epsilon Phi basketball court. I was 21, shirtless, and shooting baskets. I was too intimidated to strike up a conversation with someone so pretty and effervescent. She was there to deliver cookies to some of her friends that were at the house that day.

Luckily, I ran into her several months later at a local bar, and we chatted about Michael Jordan. I was impressed. I'd never talked to a girl about sports before, and Bryna knew her stuff. I wanted to ask her out on a date, but was intimidated. So I told her I'd make her a bet. I'd buy her dinner if Georgia lost to Alabama. I knew I had a chance because our football team was pretty bad that year. For the first time ever – and the only time – I hoped my Bulldogs would lose. They did, and we had our first date.

I began attending shows where she displayed her artwork, and I taught her how to play basketball. It was a great relationship except for one thing. I had always expected the toughest question in a relationship would be along the lines of "Do you love me?" or "Why do you watch Sportscenter every night?" Instead, it was "Why don't we ever talk about CF?"

It was a tough topic for me. Everything I knew about it was negative – I wasn't supposed to live past 25, most CFers were frail and sickly, and it made me feel vulnerable and sometimes, scared. I preferred to talk about my friends, the fraternity, Bryna, my parents, my plans, and anything else positive.

Bryna knew I had CF because her friend Sue (who was my friend Will's girlfriend) had told her. I wished she didn't know, but at the same time, I didn't like keeping secrets from her. I wished I had been the one to tell her. I wasn't angry with Sue. After all, she was her best friend. I just felt as though our relationship began like a football game without the star quarterback. It began in a hole. She had a lot of questions, but because I was so reluctant to discuss CF, she too became edgy whenever the subject arose.

The first time we talked at length about CF was over the phone. She began to cry, which made me feel terrible. I felt inadequate and guilty for bringing sadness to someone I loved. She pitied me, which didn't help. The times I'd pitied myself were the worst for me, pulling me down into despair. I didn't want her pity. I wanted support. I wanted her to say "Andy, I'm not worried. I know you'll defy the odds." Looking back, I never should have had the conversation over the phone. It's impersonal and you can't fully gauge someone's emotional reaction. Also, it's tough to hug someone when you're miles apart. We had the conversation several more times in person, but she was always the one to bring it up. I didn't feel comfortable talking about it. I preferred to just avoid it.

We'd been dating for a year when we broke up. It didn't have much to do with CF. However, the conversations about it didn't strengthen the relationship either. It was time for both of us to go separate ways. The day we decided to stop seeing each other was also the day Bryna told me she'd been researching CF and knew more than I did. I assume she told me because she wanted me to know how deep her feelings were for me and that she was trying to understand more about CF.

Looking back, I wish I'd been more open with her about CF. I just didn't know how. I considered it something so personal. Something that affected just me and maybe my parents. I did my best to keep it from having any role in my friendships and relationships because I didn't want it to overshadow everything else about me. But that's like saying the fact that I'm Jewish was something to hide, or the fact that I'm a sports junkie was something to hide. Those things are all part of who I am, and to deny any of them is to give a false picture of myself. I can't do anything to get rid of CF, but that doesn't mean it has to rule and/or overshadow my life. Trying to find the right balance for CF has never been easy, especially with a girlfriend in the picture.

I wrestled with similar issues when I began dating Stephanie, a friend of a friend. Would you believe that the first time we spent time together was at the supermarket? It takes a pretty amazing woman to get me to go to the grocery store – especially on a Saturday at midnight. We discovered we had similar interests and began dating a few months prior to my graduation from Georgia.

You'd think I would have learned something about dealing with CF from my relationship with Bryna, but I made some of the same mistakes again. The biggest being sidestepping the topic for too long. As a result, someone else told Stephanie I had CF. Of course, she was upset – but it was hard to determine if she was upset because of my CF or because I hadn't been trusting and open enough to share with her. I hadn't wanted to tell her. I feared she would have the same reaction as Bryna and I wasn't prepared to deal with more tears.

We talked about my CF in depth. And yes, Stephanie cried. What I didn't realize then was that she was crying, in part, because she was concerned about me.

I thought that conversation would be the first and last one we'd have about CF. Then we could go on in a "normal" relationship, one that involved fraternity parties, sorority functions, spring break, and movies. But Stephanie kept bringing up CF and I kept dodging her questions. Sometimes I'd fake being asleep or claim I was too tired to talk. Sometimes I'd even use CF as an excuse not to talk about CF, saying I wasn't feeling well enough then. That really upset her.

It came down to this: Despite my repeated success overcoming the limitations imposed by CF, I couldn't think of anything positive to say about a potentially fatal disease. And if I couldn't think of anything positive to say, I sure as heck wasn't going to say anything. I wasn't willing to admit that I was afraid that if she knew too much about CF, she'd see my vulnerability and then treat me differently. I wanted her to admire me. Respect me. Adore me. I thought if she knew the truth about me, she'd run.

My closed lips may have sounded like a reasonable plan, but it didn't work, thank goodness. You can't have a relationship where there's a big, glaring issue that both people have to tiptoe around. So one night, I just exploded. I poured my heart out to Stephanie. I unleashed everything I'd kept bottled up inside for years and years.

I told her that I probably couldn't have children. I told her how I was mercilessly bullied as a kid and how my parents feared for my health. I even told her about the hardest time of my life, those many months when I sunk so low that I wanted to die. I confessed that I'd hidden my therapy machine and medicines the first time she came over. I told her about how many people were unnerved by CF and how sometimes it unnerved even me. We talked for hours. Or, I should say, I talked and she listened. I cried that night as I had cried during those dark, isolated nights of my sophomore year. This time for sure, I was afraid that once she knew the "true me," she'd be out the door. But she wasn't. The opposite happened. The honesty helped bind us. It strengthened the amount of trust between us.

After that conversation, our relationship changed for the better. I changed too. I showed Stephanie my therapy machine and medicines and told her about my doctors' appointments. It was awkward at first, but the more I talked about these things that were part of my life, the easier it became for both of us. The topic was no longer taboo, so she relaxed too, which made me more comfortable talking to her. One day I even shared with her my dream of defeating CF forever. I knew she'd nod and hug me, which was just what I needed.

Sometimes I wondered if she ever thought, "Why am I with this guy?" It took me a while to realize she loved me as much as I loved her. CF just happened to be part of the whole Andy Lipman package. Stephanie helped me realize I didn't have to hide CF from anyone. And more importantly, I didn't have to hide from CF.

We dated for about two years before breaking up. It had less to do with distance – she had moved back to her hometown of Dallas to become a kindergarten teacher – than fear. Ultimately, at that point in my life, though I was healthy and optimistic about my future, I was afraid to make a commitment to her because I was afraid I couldn't fulfill it. When I got to thinking about her and us, I knew I couldn't guarantee her a long life together. I couldn't guarantee that we'd be able to have children, and I knew from the career she'd chosen that kids were important to her.

I learned a lot from Stephanie. She made me realize that I had nothing to be ashamed of because I had CF and maybe it was time that I learned more about it. And there was a lot to learn. I discovered that when I took "the test."

22

THE TEST

Fall 1999 – Age 26

In my family, it was next to impossible to get straight answers to tough questions. So after a while, I just stopped asking them. I still thought about them, particularly the mystery of my life expectancy, but I kept them to myself. I thought of my myriad questions like quicksand – they looked safe, but I knew they'd suck me under and suffocate me if I ventured in.

I tried not to blame my folks for shunning discussions about CF. I mean, what kind of parent wants to tell their child, "Yes, dear, your life expectancy is 25 so you'd better enjoy life while you can?" And what kid should have to ask, "Mom, how long am I going to live?" In my family, the way we dealt with CF was by not dealing with it. These questions chewed away at my guts, but I knew I couldn't bring them up with Mom or Dad.

Queries about the potential of sterility were also off-limits. I knew that the chances that I could have kids were about 1 in 50. I paid some attention in all those math classes – that's a piddly 2 percent. I should've been relieved. That meant I had almost nothing to worry about when the discussions on "unplanned pregnancy" rolled around before a girl and I became intimate. I figured I wouldn't ever be the subject of one of those after-school specials about the deadbeat teenage father and his impoverished infants. But I still wanted to talk to someone about this stuff.

Fertility just isn't the topic you broach with your buds. In college, the last thing you wanted to think about was impregnating someone. Well, maybe it's the first thing you think about, but you figure out pretty quickly how not to become a dad. For us, fatherhood seemed distant, something that went along with serious stuff like mortgages and car payments and an office cubicle. The biggest worries for most of my friends were who would buy the beer for that weekend's party and whether they'd pass the next business management exam. They might be sympathetic – "Oh, man, that sucks!" – but I didn't really expect them to understand.

So a year after I graduated from Georgia, I voiced my questions and concerns to Dr. Cohen. He'd been my doctor for more than a year, and he was a good guy. He never treated me like I was just his patient. He always remembered to ask me about my tennis game, and after he listened to my heart, he'd make me clench my fist. He'd give my biceps a squeeze and pretend to wince in pain. If I had an older brother, he'd probably have been like that. Dr. Cohen once told me, "You're the only patient I have who could actually kick my butt." I don't know who was more pleased by that, him or me.

But even with that kind of rapport, it wasn't easy to ask. I wanted answers, but I was afraid of them. Because once you know the truth, you lose something to hope for. It's like the families of POWs; years and years after they've vanished, their families still keep wishing and refusing to believe. They don't accept the reality until they see some bone shards or a battered, rusty dog tag. And even then, some will not be convinced. It's the only way they can keep that equilibrium they created. I was pretty comfortable with my equilibrium. Probably too comfortable. So I decided that at my next check-up, I'd change the batting order and bring Dr. Cohen to the plate. Then I'd throw him my fastball.

"There's something I need to know, but… I don't know how to ask," I told him. I knew exactly what I'd say, but I could feel my heart pulsing in my neck and in my wrists and in my head. My right foot began shaking, my nervous tic.

Dr. Cohen didn't seem to notice. "Let me guess," he said, clicking his ballpoint pen closed and clipping it onto my file. "You want to know how long you're going to live."

Maybe they teach mind reading in medical school. "Yeah," I said. "I want to know how long I'm going to live." I'd said the words to myself for so long that they sounded perfectly mundane, as though I'd asked for a Coke. But I felt defiant, like I was daring him to punch me as hard as he could.

I watched his face for pity or sympathy, but his familiar attentive expression didn't change. He didn't seem to be someone ready to announce somber news.

"Honestly, Andy, you can live into your 70s or 80s," he said, looking into my eyes. "If you stay in shape and have a little luck along the way, you're here for the long haul."

It felt like the truth, and not just because that's what I so desperately wanted to hear. As soon as he said "the long haul," I felt lighter. It was the way you feel when you're bench-pressing 250 pounds and you slide off 50 pounds and get back on the bench. The bar that was ready to crush your neck feels no heavier than a broom, and you're good for a dozen more quick reps. I'd been lugging around my question for years, and I didn't know how much it was weighing me down, how much it sucked up my strength. I realized I was still breathing, and I thought: Man, you'll be breathing this fine air for the next 50, 60 years. I was on a roll.

"O.K., what are my chances of having children?"

Dr. Cohen paused and then said, "Andy, you have a better chance than most."

That I knew wasn't true. But I never expected him to lie.

"Look," I said, "I know there's a 2 percent chance. You know it. You don't have to sugar-coat it."

He glanced down for a second and ran his thumb along the crease of my folder.

"Gotcha," I thought.

"I'm not sugar-coating anything. You've taken good care of yourself. You're in better shape than most people. I'd say your chances are about 50-50."

"Really?" Another reprieve. Fifty-fifty wasn't bad at all, and it was a heck of a lot better than I'd trained myself to think. I could see myself jogging through Piedmont Park with one of those three-wheeled strollers or teaching my kid how to sink a basket. But I didn't want to get my hopes up. I get that fine strain of pessimism from Aunt Susie, my favorite cynic. There was a 75 percent chance I wouldn't get CF, but, hey, I got it. Fifty-fifty might not be much better.

"But you can find out for sure," Dr. Cohen said. "There's a lab that can tell you. I'll get you the number."

He did, but I didn't call. The number sat on my desk for weeks, reminding me that just because I could find out the answer to a question didn't mean I had to. I might never have called if it hadn't been for Stephanie.

"Met anyone?" she asked, with candor that only old girlfriends have.

Yes and no, I told her. Had a date with a girl who smoked. Forget it. Went out with a gorgeous woman with a mouth like a sailor. Got fixed up with a girl who was so shy she made even me uncomfortable. Had a couple dates with perfectly nice women, but we just didn't click. There was something wrong with every one.

Or...there was something wrong with me. I was so quick to pick everyone apart so I could write them off. Because it's easier to be the one doing the rejecting than the one who's rejected. And if they never get to know me, they'd never discover that I have CF or that I might be sterile. So they'd never dump me because they wanted a husband for the long haul or a man who could be a father. I needed to give someone a chance to get to know me. And if she truly loved me then we could work around the CF and make the relationship work. I didn't tell this to Stephanie, though. I'd just figured it out myself.

I think you can lie to yourself for only so long. So the next day, I called the clinic. The receptionist very matter-of-factly told me to be abstinent for two days and then to "produce" a sperm specimen and drop it off before it was more than an hour old. I was lucky on both counts: I lived near the office, and the abstinence issue, unfortunately, was a done deal. So I went by the office and dropped off the sample. It wouldn't be long before I found out the answer.

23

THE ANSWER

Fall 1999 – Age 26

The ideal way to find out whether or not you'll be able to have children is not by a doctor's e-mailed note. I advise against this. But when it shows up in your "in" box, what can you do? I guess I could've waited until I went home to read it. Yeah, right.

Dr. Cohen apologized for not calling me, explaining that he was out of town. He knew I was eager for the results of the test, though, so his note got right to the point. My sperm sample, he wrote, was "sub-optimal" which probably meant that it wasn't up to the task of fertilizing an egg. In other words, I'm shooting blanks. I'm not going to be able to have kids, at least not the way most people do.

This shouldn't be a big surprise to me. I knew that 98 percent of men with CF are sterile because most have a blocked vas deferens, which carries the sperm from the testicles to the penis. But I still couldn't give up the hope, and I felt cheated, somehow. I'd overcome so many obstacles that CF had put in front of me that fertility somehow seemed manageable too.

Prior to the test, I told myself that whether or not I could father a child shouldn't matter. I told myself that one day I'm going to find a girl who will love me for who I am. She will love the way I make her laugh, and she will love the fact that I'm her best friend. She'll think I'm handsome, smart, cool, and a little goofy. If she's the love of my life, how much will she care about "sub-optimal" sperm?

I took heart from something that Stephanie said when she called, hours after I was mulling over the test results and how they'd affect my life down the line. She said, "When we were dating, I always knew you couldn't have children, but, you know, I wanted to be with you anyway." Surely she couldn't be the only one.

That afternoon I went to lunch with my dad, Aunt Susie, and Renae, my dad's administrative assistant. Renae joked, "Let's worry first about finding you a girlfriend." You know, she's right. It's not like I've got a biological clock ticking or anything. I'm a 26-year-old guy. Right now, I'm not in any rush to take Lamaze classes and change dirty diapers (I don't think I'll ever be rushing to do that, to be honest). My renewed perspective cheered me up, at least for a little while.

Then Aunt Susie suggested adoption. Thanks to my younger sister Emily, I knew plenty about adoption. I wondered if agencies would be reluctant to place a baby with my wife (whoever she may be) and myself because of my CF. They might fear that my life expectancy and medical issues would create problems. I'd hope CF wouldn't defer an adoption because, to be honest, no one knows how much time he or she has. Anyone could be stricken by anything at any time, be it cancer or a car accident. The way I look at it, CF is at least a known quantity. I only wish I didn't know it quite so well.

That night, however, when I got home, I cried. Strangely, it was with a more tempered kind of anger and frustration than I'd had before. If I'd gotten the same results about fertility while still in college, it might have been just enough to push me over the edge – and possibly take my own life.

Now, though, I've toughened up to CF. After years, it has become a known quantity, like a pitcher on an opposing team. Once you get to know his fastball and his curveball, you're better prepared for whatever he throws. He can't fake you out anymore. I'll take an enemy I know over one that I don't.

I began reading about other ways to have children. One such method was Microscopic Epididyum/Sperm Aspiration (MESA) in which semen would be collected from my testicles (via a needle) and then comined in a laboratory dish with a woman's eggs to see if fertilization could occur. The results were mixed, but it was still a potential option.

But there was still the matter of finding someone who

would love me and accept some of the limitations posed by CF. Someone who believed that I could accomplish anything. Alas, I found her.

24

MEETING SOMEONE NEW: CF'S NO LONGER TABOO

Spring 1999 – Age 25

During the years after Stephanie and I broke up, I remained in Atlanta for work and I dated a lot. Nothing special, really, but good practice in meeting girls and being myself. I began mentioning CF earlier when I was in a relationship. I wasn't afraid to bring it up even on the first date, though I now realize that wasn't always the best approach. There's nothing like the revelation that your date has a fatal disorder to turn a promising evening into a polite handshake and "Thanks, I had a really nice time. Bye."

As positive as I am about my life and my experience with CF, other people aren't always as knowledgeable or accepting, and sometimes their ignorance gets in the way. I can't control that, unfortunately. I once had a girl back out of a date with me because previously, I'd been so sick that I had to cancel. She knew I had CF, and I couldn't help but think that she was afraid I already had a foot in the grave. Our first three dates were pretty nice I thought, but it was probably tough to foresee a future with me when I had to cancel the fourth date because I could hardly breathe. I remembered the girl in college who freaked out when she saw me doing my therapy. I'd seen the worst in people, who didn't understand CF, but thanks to people like Bryna and Stephanie, I knew there was a lot of good as well.

Which brings me to Andrea. I met her at a birthday party and was immediately struck by her smile, which made the most spectacular sunset pale in comparison. I felt a spark the moment she walked into the courtyard. But there was a lot more to Andrea than her beauty. She was smart – a master's degree from Emory University and a nimble mind that could win a debate with any politician – and (thank you, God) athletic. She played football, softball, ran track, and swam.

We didn't get much past "Oh, hi" at the party, but I couldn't forget her. Luckily, I didn't have to. Several weeks later, a friend called to ask if I'd be willing to talk to Andrea, who was going through a tough time with thyroid cancer. My friend thought my experiences in battling CF might help Andrea with her problem. "Glad to help," I said, telling myself that I was simply being a pal and had no ulterior motives whatsoever.

So Andrea and I discussed her problem over a really nice lunch. We talked about our resentment of hospitals and our need for people to be there for us. She said she felt better – I know I did! – and before long we were talking every day. It just seemed natural to tell her about my problems with CF, which at the time were worse than usual because I was really sick. She didn't seem bothered at all. If I had told anyone else I coughed up phlegm all the time, that person would wrinkle their nose and say "Gross." Andrea, though, would ask, "What did the doctor prescribe? Is there a treatment you can do?" It was an added bonus that she was knowledgeable about CF – she worked for the Center for Disease Control and Prevention.

After only one day of knowing Andrea, I felt comfortable enough to give her the manuscript for this book. Basically, I laid my life story in her hands. I figured if she was going to take off, she'd at least be able to do it fast and no one would get hurt. But she stuck around in a big way. And her reaction was like no one else's had ever been. She said: "Don't let cystic fibrosis consume you. It's just a disease. It's not you."

I was smitten, but Andrea didn't want to date me. She was very kind when she explained that she thought I was a really good friend and a great guy, but she was busy with other things in her life and wasn't looking for a relationship. My friends told me to give up and move on. Aunt Susie told me that Andrea was a terrific person, but she and I were just not meant for each other. My roommate, Ross, who became my closest friend after college, was concerned that I was in the market for a "Reject" sign to paste on my forehead.

It was CF, ironically, that lent a helping hand. CF had always taught me to never give up, even when people were doubtful I would succeed. If I believed in myself, then I could accomplish what other people thought was unattainable. I learned to never give up on my dreams, and Andrea was certainly a dream of mine. It took a year, but Andrea and I risked our incredible friendship and began to date.

We'd been together for a few months when one night on the way home from a date we plunged into the infamous "CF Discussion." I knew it so well I could have practically prompted Andrea on her lines. It went something like this:

"Andy, I've been thinking about the fact that you probably can't have kids and that you have CF. It's scary," she said. (Cue mournful violin music.) "I've been thinking about it for a long time."

I knew where this was headed. I standing at the Greyhound station with a suitcase and a one-way ticket to a map-dot town called Breakup City.

But Andrea surprised me. She squeezed my hand, grinned, and said, "I'm comfortable with things. I am cool with adopting. Whatever happens, I'm happy just being with you."

Whoa. Say what? "So you're saying …" I couldn't even finish the sentence.

"Andy, isn't it obvious? I love you," she said. (Chirping birds and soaring orchestra. Dancing gnomes.)

Man oh man. I'd told her two weeks earlier I loved

her, but I was worried she didn't feel the same way about me. And the fact that she did – unbelievable, amazing, wonderful, and heavenly all at the same time!

Andrea continues to stun me. She's so cool. I didn't mention that she loves to travel. I mean really travel, not just go to Savannah for a weekend or visit Disneyworld. She likes to explore the world. She knew I had to use my chest therapy machine, which, though it's portable, isn't something you could stuff in a backpack while hiking the Scottish moors. So she was thrilled to learn that I didn't have to lug it with me – as long as someone could administer my therapy. Right then and there she volunteered to learn how to do it. So my mom taught her. I am in love with this girl. Talk about a unique bonding experience. Earlier in my life I felt trapped because my parents had to administer my therapy, but now I was more secure with my future. I had met someone who cared about me and who wanted to make it easier for me to travel. So it was okay if she wanted to pound on my chest every now and then.

Andrea still worried when I got even the mildest of colds, but I understood that. It helped to remind her that many CFers were living well into their 40s and 50s and beyond with CF. She didn't know that. Then again, not many people did, which was one reason I wanted to write this book.

I couldn't help but think I'd finally found the girl from my dreams. The one who I saw in the department store. The one who asked me if I needed any help. The girl, who like Andrea, had brown hair and brown eyes. Still I was not attracted to the girl in the dream and Andrea was beautiful in my eyes. I guess she couldn't be the girl from the dream, but if it wasn't her, who was it?

Andrea and I have been dating for well over a year, and I couldn't be happier. I realize we probably wouldn't be dating at all if I hadn't adjusted my attitude about CF. I've finally developed a mindset that I lacked with Bryna and Stephanie. My mindset before I dated Andrea was that I'd be lucky to find anyone to date me because after all, I was going to die young and was unable to have children. So why would someone want me? Obviously, this line of thinking did wonders for my self-esteem.

My attitude turned around thanks to a combination of things. I spent some time with a therapist, who helped me honestly examine my accomplishments and give myself credit for what I've done, how I'm living my life, and my many positive attributes. I began to realize that any girl would be lucky to have me, and I had a right to be picky, too. That wasn't arrogance – I still thought Christie Brinkley wouldn't be returning my calls any time soon – but self-assurance.

For a long time, I blamed my relationship problems on CF. Granted, it's not easy finding someone when you have a disease like cystic fibrosis. Now, however, I see it differently: Once you've found someone who can live with you and your CF, you have found someone truly special. I've also learned that it's important to be honest about CF. Not simply that I have it now and I'll always have it, but that it's a part of who I am. Denying that is denying who I am.

Before, when someone asked me how I was doing, I'd say only "Fine" or "O.K." and wouldn't elaborate. I didn't think anyone would be interested in what I had to say. But now I'd realized how wrong that was. Most people asked because they genuinely cared. Telling them just "O.K." didn't bring us any closer. It was painful to open up, but with the right people, it was worth it. Especially when something important came up. And when I was defying the odds on the athletic fields, there was nothing more important.

25

ATHLETICS: MY WAY OF COPING

Spring 1999 – Age 25

When I first read the encyclopedia article about CF that said my days were numbered, I didn't know what to do. When a big, authoritative book bluntly tells you you're not going to make it past 25, it's hard to ignore that and get on with your life. I didn't have much else to go on. Kids asked if I was going to die – and why would they ask unless they thought I wasn't going to make it? – and the only movie I'd seen about CF involved a girl who became a victim. Giving up seemed to be the only option.

Sports, however, sent me the opposite message. Competition taught me that the harder I worked, the better I became. And there was plenty of room for improvement. I was always the last person picked for baseball teams in gym class. I knew I had very little stamina and I couldn't catch or throw. The only thing I knew how to do was dream. This was my dream: One day I'd stroll onto the field and members of the opposing team would take notice. With their voices lowered in whispers of respect, they'd say, "That's the MVP" – the most valuable player on the team.

That fantasy became a reality when I was, fittingly enough, 25. I led my team in hits, runs, at-bats, games played, and scraped knees from hustling from one base to the next. I was in the top two in home runs, batting average, triples, and runs batted in. My teammates, the people who really knew how I played, chose me as the MVP. I received a foot-high trophy with my name and the team's name on it. I'm proud of that trophy and it's displayed on my bookshelf at home.

Few of my teammates knew I had CF, and I liked to keep it that way. I wanted them to say "Great play!" when I slid into home plate – not "Great play for someone who has CF." I also tried to be supportive of other players because I remembered very clearly how it felt to be mocked and shunned in Little League. My teammates called me "Sunny" because I saw the "sunny" side of any situation. I was the first to compliment people on how they played regardless of the score of the game. I knew how good a word of support or appreciation made me feel, and I wanted to do that for others as well.

I liked softball so much that I played on five teams that season. I gave each of them all I had. And the more I gave, the more I had. When a ball slipped past me in practice, I would ask the batter to hit another one to me, even harder. When I made an error, I tried to improve on it with a better play. I was proving something to myself and I was proving something about CF – it couldn't stop me.

It tried, though, several times. One particular episode was during a basketball game that year. We'd been playing for three hours. The game was tied, and each side desperately wanted the winning point. I began coughing violently and nearly doubled over on the court. One of the players on the other team laughed and said, "Looks like we found the smoker in the group!" All my life, strangers who hear my wrenching cough have never hesitated to offer all sorts of unsolicited advice about quitting smoking or going to see a doctor. Gee, thanks.

A player on the other team took a shot and missed the basket. I grabbed the ball, ran down the court, made the basket, and won the game. Then I fell to the ground and heaved up a big wad of phlegm. Not a pretty sight, but I'd bet they thought it was darn good for a pack-a-day smoker!

I had another sports victory at the gym that year. I'd been working out with a personal trainer who really pushed me to excel. (As I've said, the more I'm challenged, the better I do.) I'd been feeling really good, especially after a great visit to the doctor and a new nutrition plan from my trainer. One afternoon at the gym I lifted 275 pounds a few times. I wasn't tired. I realized I might be able to reach my goal and lift 300.

That goal was born in college, when most of the stronger guys in the fraternity said it was their aim. I could barely lift 105 pounds at the time, and 300 seemed totally out of reach – until that day. I slid weights totaling 305 pounds onto the bar. I then glanced around the gym for someone to spot me on this massive lift when, from out of nowhere, I saw Donald*.

He was the same guy who 12 years earlier had bullied me in the cafeteria at Peachtree High School by pushing my books onto the floor, dumping my lunch into the garbage, and then laughing in my face. It still stung when I remembered how other kids laughed with him – at me. I might as well have been wearing a shirt that said, "Ridicule me, please. And if it's not too much trouble, beat me up as soon as possible."

My grades and my confidence both slipped. My mom knew something was wrong, but I wouldn't share with her. It was my battle, and I was going to have to fight it myself. I felt so frustrated. That frustration built until one day when Donald tried to grab my lunch. I shouted "No!" He pushed me. "Give it to me," he demanded. Then he saw the principal coming and pretended to stroll away. But after that, he stopped bothering me.

That experience made me realize that bullies seek out easy victims, the ones who don't fight back. I had plenty of experience battling CF, and in the big picture, Donald wasn't so terrifying. Still, you never forget the feeling of being humiliated, no matter how much time passes. I couldn't forget Donald, and when he saw me at the gym, it was obvious he hadn't forgotten me either.

"Andy?" he said. "You're a lot bigger." His eyes were staring as if he was still coming to grips with the fact that this was the same kid in high school that he used to push around. "Hey, man, I'm sorry about what happened, you know, when we were kids."

"No big deal," I said with a shrug. "I barely remember it. Spot me?"

"Sure."

We walked over to the bench together and I could see him adding up the pounds in his head. "This is over 300," he said, looking at me for the first time with a little fear and a hint of respect.

"Really?" I wanted to give him the impression I did this all the time.

I settled onto my back on the bench, gripped the barbell, and took a few deep breaths. Wait a minute...how the heck was I going to lift all this weight?

I lifted the same way I blew those pulmonary function tests. I willed every ounce of energy I had into my muscles and slowly, strongly raised the barbell into the air. Beads of sweat ran down my face. I lowered the bar onto the rack. Before I had a chance to soak up Donald's astonishment, I glanced over at the man on the equipment next to me. He was obviously dressed for my performance. His T-shirt read, "Join the CF team." I was already a member, but I was ready to lead the team to victory.

I lifted weights with Donald for a couple of months, and I never told him I had CF. I didn't want his pity. And I didn't want him to feel even worse about mistreating me in school. I just wanted his respect, and it was clear I had gotten it.

At different times in my life, people like Donald, Uncle Bobby, and my basketball adversary, Brett had all personified the challenges of CF to me, but the biggest doubter was clearly me. I was the one who often second-guessed my abilities and downplayed my achievements.

I've trained myself over the last couple of years to lessen my pessimistic ways. When I have a moment of doubt about CF, I repeat a sentence in my head again and again. It's what you might call a mantra, and it's an acronym for cystic fibrosis. When there are two outs in the final inning of a tied softball game or there is a tense moment on the job, I will tell myself: Can't You See That I Can Fight It, But Remember Only Strong Individuals Survive.

It works for me, and I'd like to share that with other CFers. Some have been coping with this enemy for a lot longer than I have. I've read about people in their 40s, 50s, and 60s with CF. Though not everyone is as athletic as I am, they are all survivors, people who laugh in the face of CF and every day prove that CF encyclopedia article wrong.

One of my regrets for so many years, however, was that I'd never known any of these fellow soldiers. I'd never had any type of relationship with anyone with CF. Would I ever get the chance?

26
END OF ISOLATION

Summer 1999 – Age 25

I'd always wondered what it would be like to have a friend who understood me completely. It's not that I didn't have friends. I'd had buddies as addicted to sports and fitness as I was, and I'd had a gaggle of college friends and fraternity brothers who agonized over the same exams and girls as I did.

But I'd never had friends who understood all that...plus CF. They could only imagine what it was like to know they couldn't have children or to have to take pills with every meal. They would never experience the embarrassment of heaving up a chunk of phlegm as people watched in disgust, assuming it was uncouth manners or some type of plague taking its toll. And they'd never read an article about their life expectancy. Of course, doctors who specialized in CF knew about the symptoms, related risks, and medications that went along with the disease, but again, that's not the same as living with it. That's something only fellow CFers knew and I didn't know any CFers.

One of the ironies of CF is that the people I'd most like to meet – other CFers – are pretty much off-limits. We each carry zillions of bacteria and, unfortunately, run a big risk of infecting each other with whatever it is that we don't have. It's scary because two people with CF can do serious harm to each other without ever intending to. Thus, it's critical that we keep our distance. The situation is the antithesis of a leper colony, where people with leprosy were quarantined together in "colonies" or even on a Hawaiian island to protect everyone else, not them.

I found my link to CFers the same way that everyone from Model T enthusiasts to pumpkin growers hook up these days: through the Internet. I clicked on the Website www.esiason.org, which was created by former Monday Night Football announcer Boomer Esiason, whose son, Gunnar, has CF. What immediately caught my attention were the profiles of CFers who were living normal, exciting lives.

I was especially inspired by Jason, a guy who played sports, lifted weights, and worked for the Charlotte Hornets basketball team. I read his profile and looked up his phone number. I called him, despite my doubts about getting in touch. I thought that like me sometimes, he might not want to talk about CF. But I figured I had nothing to lose.

When he answered the phone, I noticed immediately that he sounded great – no gasping for air or wheezing like the CFers I'd read about. We hit it off immediately and talked about everything from my infertility to who the Hornets were going to play the next season. He was the first CFer I talked to about topics besides CF. Then again, besides Chris, the boy who came over to examine my therapy machine when I was a teenager, he was the only CFer I'd ever talked to. Since that first phone call, we've e-mailed each other every now and then to share stories, fears, and hopes. For so long, when I thought of a CFer, I thought of someone like Chris: frail, thin, and hoarse from coughing. I also couldn't forget the other people with CF I saw in doctors' offices. They needed someone to help them across the room, and many were connected to a network of tubes. The only movie I'd seen about CF featured a kid who died at age 8, and the only material I'd read about CF said I'd be dead by 25.

Talking with Jason and just knowing he was out there, living a life he loved, and feeling good was exactly what I needed. It gave me hope and it inspired me, and I told him so. Jason seemed surprised.

"It's funny," he said. "I never think of myself as inspiring anyone. I just try to live my life to the best of my ability."

That's what I'd say, too. I remember when my friend Seth asked how I was doing, I said, "Oh, I'm getting by."

He laughed and said, "For you, getting by is what

most people would consider overachieving."

I figured I was on a roll, so I also called Kathy, another person featured on the Esiason Website. She's an all-star hockey player for Northeastern University in Boston and has been on "Good Morning America" and in Sports Illustrated. We talked about how a sense of humor can help keep CF in perspective and how friends' jokes about coughing and other symptoms are actually welcome because they make us feel accepted. We agreed that it's best for us to ignore the news updates about possible cures for CF. We've been hearing the same thing since we were kids and nothing's happened yet. You have to be optimistic that one day there will be a cure, we agreed, but you have to keep taking care of yourself in the meantime.

I thought Kathy was a huge inspiration, and I felt like she was doing me a big favor by sharing her experiences with me. Then I got this e-mail:

"After our conversation, I spent another full hour telling my roommates how inspirational you are and how excited it made me to know that there are others out there like me. This surprised me because you had the same feelings, fears and thoughts that I had! I always thought I was the only one!"

Speaking with Jason and Kathy led me to an Internet chat room for CFers and their families called the Cystic-L. Soon I was getting dozens of e-mails each day with questions about everything from medications to insurance. It was a great way to connect with others and share positive energy. Some of the most inspiring messages came from people in their 50s with CF – and even a 68-year-old guy. There were people out there living long lives with CF. That's what I liked to hear.

I didn't expect negative stuff, too, but that was there as well. Some people wrote, "I don't think I can fight it anymore" and even "I wish my parents had never had me." I'd been e-mailing a woman named Alisa who was going into the hospital for surgery. She wrote back afterward to say she hurt, but was going to be O.K. She was always the person who supported my positive approach to CF. She was as tough as nails. She died the next day. That really shook me. I couldn't help but mourn a woman I'd only written to a couple of times, someone who was part of my extended CF family.

It was this aspect of the chat room that disturbed my dad. He thought that it attracted people who were needy or who were negative, not the ones who were busy living fulfilled lives. I know he was afraid negative comments and cold realities like Alisa's death would bring me down, and to some degree, they did. That's reality. That's life with CF. But for me, the benefits outweighed the negative stuff.

One of the most important things the CF chat room did was dispel my stereotype of CFers. I know I should be the last one to stereotype anyone with CF, but hey, I admit I did. Getting in touch with a variety of people with CF made me realize that we come in all varieties. Sure, some people were sickly, but many, like Jason and

Kathy, were healthy, active, and optimistic.

I found one of my best friends through the CF chat room. I've never met Michelle, who lives in Nebraska, but we clicked immediately. I wish we could have lived in the same city – though I don't know if my Southern-born body could handle those bitter winters – but because of the risks of two people with CF being in the same room, I know we'll always be apart.

Michelle loves to hike, and her goal is to climb down and then back up the Grand Canyon, just to prove that someone with CF can do it. I love that atti-tude. I understand it so well. It's the same mindset I had when I stepped up to bat or paused for that split second before making a jump shot. We seemed to comprehend each other perfectly, and I wondered if maybe Michelle has been the girl in my dream...in the shopping mall asking if I need help. She's certainly been a huge com-fort and help.

We've found that we have so much in common. Her father has as hard a time dealing with CF as my mom does. Both feel very protective of us and neither likes to accompany us on doctors' appointments. They love us so much and don't want to see us in any pain. It's as if Michelle and I lived parallel lives.

I still dream about meeting her one day. I think we can't be too far away from a test that would detect if people with CF carried anything that was dangerously contagious. Once we knew we were both O.K., we'd plan to finally get together. We'd do it on "Oprah," maybe. Why not? It wouldn't hurt the world to see two happy, healthy people who just happen to have CF. I hope that day isn't too far away, that one day everyone with CF could get together. Maybe in Las Vegas. Again, why not?

I probably wouldn't have "met" her if we each didn't have CF. Clearly, I wish we didn't have CF, but then again, who knows how different our lives would have otherwise been? Sometimes the biggest frustrations and disappointments in our lives can also turn out to be the biggest blessings. I think it's a matter of being grateful for what you do have and focusing on the positive, rather than obsessing on the negative.

Michelle and I still talk over the phone and e-mail and we've been doing that for over two years. We have gotten each other through some tough times. And guess what? Michelle is now engaged to her boyfriend of over a year, Joe. I'm happy because he really treats her well. It's a good thing because I wouldn't accept anything but the best for Michelle. By the way, she may be inviting Andrea and I to the wedding. So June of 2002, barring any bacterial infections, may be the time we finally meet face-to-face and it was CF that brought us together.

So I hold tight to the group of friends from all over the country that I've made over the CF chat line. They strengthen me as much as I strengthen them. That's real friendship. Their companionship has ended my CF-induced isolation. I know I can turn to them for support, advice, and good humor. My life feels pretty complete.

Except for the girl in the mall. She's not Michelle. I know that, though I'm not sure how. I need to find out who she is.

27

MORE THAN A NAME

Spring 1999 – Age 25

While writing this book, I wanted to talk to my mom about my life. There were so many things I wanted to know, but I didn't want to upset her. I think by asking her to relive the sometimes painful details about my struggles as a young CFer or by asking her outright about her fears about me, my health, and my life, I'm hurting her. I'm sure she thinks a lot about that type of stuff. It comes with the territory of being a mom, especially the mom of a CFer. And though I'm now an adult, I'll always be her child.

But to be honest, it was more than just about my mom. It was me as well. It was tough for me to have a candid conversation with my mom. I think I got that from my dad. He said he deals with my CF by basically staying in denial – by not pondering what'll happen to me other than what's happening today. It works for

him, and it works for me. At least, it worked for me
until I began writing this book. Writing broadened my
perspective and made me realize that I didn't know my
mom very well and I wanted to know more. I felt self-
conscious asking her, and a little intrusive. If she'd
wanted me to know, wouldn't she have told me? But I
asked anyway.

The best way to learn more, I thought, was to read
sections of this book to her as I wrote them and then
wait for her response. So I called her and asked her to
listen to what I'd written so far. "Sure," she said. I started at the beginning: "I was born at Northside Hospital
in Atlanta and weighed 10 pounds, 10 ounces."

Mom interrupted me to gush: "You were the biggest
baby in the hospital that day! Did you know that? You
were a giant!"

"I know, Ma, I know," I said, pretending exasperation, but secretly, I loved it. Mom always bragged about
what a hefty infant I was, as though it was a sign that
I'd be a formidable fighter against CF and a strong athlete. My birth weight had attained the status of family
legend.

I continued: "I was due in August 1973, but I was
born a month late."

Mom laughed. I knew what she was going to say,
and she didn't disappoint me. "The doctors thought
you would never pop out," she said with a chuckle.

"I know, I know," I said. "It's your fault for having
me on Labor Day. Get it, Mom?"

Now it was her turn to pretend to be exasperated. "Yes, Andy, very funny."

I turned serious and continued: "As you can see, I have a lousy sense of humor and an excuse for every-thing – everything except cystic fibrosis. The fact that I was born with such a dangerous, even deadly illness must have been very hard on my parents, who lost their first child two years earlier."

I paused so the words could settle.

"Is it O.K. if I mention that?" I asked.

"Yes, that's fine," Mom softly replied.

What I'd written was pretty much everything I knew about Wendy, my older sister. Her birthday was December 18th. I knew that. I also knew she lived just a few days. I assumed she died from Sudden Infant Death Syndrome or something similar, but I really did-n't know. I'd always wanted to know more, but I could sense her short life was a painful topic for my parents. Not wanting to upset them, I kept my questions about Wendy to a minimum. I knew I gave them enough to worry about. Sometimes in mid-December, my mom would tell me, out of the blue, "You know, you're lucky to be alive."

That little statement left me with a pang of guilt, a sense that I had been coasting through my life, grum-bling about little stuff and missing the big picture. But the reminder left me feeling bitter, as though I needed a jolt to re-ignite my sense of gratitude. Whenever my mom said it, I had a hunch she was thinking of Wendy, of lost opportunities, of missed chances. I always thought of anything that had to do with Wendy as a blanket of sorrow woven with threads of guilt, grief, and silence.

I felt emboldened by my book project, and I decided I wouldn't wrap that blanket around me like my parents had done. In my mind, I shook it out, folded it up, and asked: "Mom, tell me how Wendy died."

Suddenly, right there, I thought of a possibility I'd either been blind to or willfully ignorant of: "Was it CF?"

Now I wasn't sure I wanted to know. I could hear my mom's breath catch, and I knew she was forced to look once again into a room whose door she'd done her best to shut.

"Yes, Andy, it was CF," she said. Her voice was ragged and she started crying.

Usually, that sound alone would stop me because I hate upsetting my mother. This time, though, that tiny bit of information was too enticing. I had to know more, even if it stung both of us. I could sense a momentous conversation approaching between me and my mom.

"What else?" I asked. I could hear the rough scrape of a tissue being pulled from a box – I knew it was the box on the kitchen counter by the clutter of bills, lists, and memos – and then the sound of my mom blowing her nose. She sighed.

"She died because she had a meconium ileus, a

blockage in her intestines," Mom said dully.

"Didn't I have that?"

"Yes, but the doctors gave you a barium enema and it worked. They also noticed the problem a lot faster with you because of what happened with Wendy."

She sighed again.

"Your father and I went through a lot with her. Oh, Andy, she was so beautiful – light brown hair and the most beautiful brown eyes."

I pictured my ecstatic mom and dad, new parents cuddling their firstborn, elated, dazed, overwhelmed, giddy, not knowing that sorrow was just days away. I felt their grief seep into my throat before lodging in my heart.

"I put flowers and a stuffed animal on her grave every year on her birthday," she said.

My mother's secret grieving ritual – something I'd never known in all the years I'd lived with her. I didn't say anything. To get my mom to talk to me about something so personal and painful was rare, and I feared she might clam up if I said the wrong thing. Maybe if I said anything.

"I would have told you, but –" Mom said, sniffling. "I wasn't sure you were ready."

"I'm sorry, Mom," I told her. "I didn't know."

When we hung up, I felt a fresh wave of empathy for my mom. Instead of strictly seeing her as an overprotective parent, I saw her as a woman who'd suffered a tremendous loss and couldn't help but fear that she might mourn another child.

When Wendy died, Mom couldn't have been much older than I was. How would I have handled that? No one's ready for death, but the death of a child – that's more than anyone should bear. No wonder she was so careful to guard me from infections and injuries, real or perceived. And how many times had I shrugged off her concern or mocked her protection? If only I'd known.

I mulled this over as I dressed for the gym and got in the car. I gradually realized I was angry, too. How could my parents shield me from the truth? Not telling me about what killed Wendy was just the same as lying, really. Why couldn't we talk about these things? Would we ever be able to?

The radio began playing "The Wind Beneath My Wings," and the lyrics made me cry, especially the line about "a beautiful face without a name." For me, Wendy was a beautiful name without a face. It wasn't until today that I knew anything about her, even something as mundane as the color of her eyes and hair.

"Wendy," I thought as I wept, "I'm sorry we never met. Your death in some ways gave me life. If it hadn't been for you, the doctors might never have noticed my condition, and I might have died, like you." That made me think about the incredibly fragile chain of coincidences, chances, and strokes of luck that brought me to this moment. Bette Midler was singing about how "you're my hero; you're everything I would like to be." I was crying so hard that I had to pull off the road.

Most of the time, the radio is pure background

noise, something to hum along to when I'm sitting in traffic or lifting weights. Yet every once in a while, a song comes on and because of what I'm thinking at that time, it becomes indelibly connected to something important in my life. That's the way it's been with this song. I must've heard it dozens, maybe even hundreds of times before then and virtually ignored it. But I knew I'd never hear it again without feeling mingled sadness and gratitude. It would remind me of Wendy, my big sister who never lived past infancy.

* * *

You might think the emotional ride to the gym would be enough for one night. I could've turned around and gone home. My eyes were red and swollen from crying, and my nose was running. Once I make up my mind to go to the gym, though, it pretty much takes a natural disaster to keep me out of the weight room. Although I looked like I'd just sat through a Hallmark made-for-TV special, I pulled into the gym and launched into my workout.

Concentration on something that was solely physical was the perfect antidote. I lost myself lifting and lowering weights, working on my form, and if the truth must be told, scoping out the cute girls in workout gear. I felt a lot better.

My last stop of the evening was the pull-up machine. I was on my last set, the toughest ones, where your body is shaking and telling you to stop and your brain is urging you to try for a few more...five...six... seven...eight...just two more!...nine...I closed my eyes and put everything I had into that last effort when suddenly that friendly, familiar face of the mysterious dream girl appeared in my head. This time, I wasn't perplexed. I knew exactly who it was. She was, of course, Wendy.

28

CEMETERY MEETING

Spring 1999 – Age 25

As far as I knew, there was nothing tangible in my parents' house to tell anyone they once had a daughter named Wendy except one hospital photo that my mom had tucked away somewhere. Aunt Susie said the photo was one of Mom's most precious possessions. I had never seen the snapshot, and I wasn't about to ask Mom to see it. I wish she'd offered, but she never did. I felt the photo was something Mom would show me when she was ready...and I wasn't going to rush that. Sometimes I wondered whether Wendy even existed, and I realized that after my parents had died, there'd be no one left who remembered anything about her. I wanted something from Wendy I could see and touch, something that said – proved, maybe? – that she had lived, however briefly.

I realized that the thing I sought did exist. It was

Wendy's grave. I knew I had to see it, but I wasn't sure why. I knew other people left stuffed animals, pictures, or flowers on graves. I didn't feel any urge to leave things for her. I just wanted to know whether the sun shone on her grave, whether it was nicely tended, and whether the little stone bore her name. Did it say "Wendy Carol Lipman, Dec. 18, 1970 – Jan. 2, 1971"?

The best way I could describe it was to say that I felt a strong need to go to the one place on earth where her name appeared and introduce myself and apologize for not visiting sooner. I felt I owed that to her because in some way, I was living the life she never had a chance to live. She knew that. She helped and protected me, sort of like a guardian angel.

I wondered if she was checking up on me when she appeared in that recurring dream I've had since I was a child. I was hiding under a clothes rack in a store; this girl who appeared to be a couple of years older than me saw me and very politely asked, "Do you need any help?" I was not at all offended that she was asking, not any more than I'd be if a salesperson asked me the same question. And that's sort of how she asked it, though I knew she was not a store employee. In my dream, I always shook my head and told her, "No." And then she vanishes, not at all miffed.

For so many years, I tried to wring some meaning out of that dream, especially since I've had it several times. My first thought was that it had something to do with being lost in the mall as a kid – but if that were the case and this nice person was offering to help me, wouldn't I have accepted her help? As I grew older, I thought maybe she was the girl I'd marry, but I didn't feel love-struck when I saw her, just comfortable. She seemed familiar and friendly. And I didn't have any physical attraction to her, which, well, made me think that maybe she was a version of my grandmother Ethel Lipman who had died of leukemia years earlier. (But I think if she had been my grandmother, she would've said, "Young man, what do you think you're doing? You get out from under that clothes rack right now!")

But if the helpful girl was Wendy, why would we meet in the mall? And why under a clothes rack? I kept turning it over in my head until I realized I was hiding from something in a big public place and looking for a haven where I felt secure. Maybe the mall was the world and the clothes rack was my own personal haven, my brain, or my room? The fact she found me so easily and didn't seem at all surprised to see me made me think she knew me well and didn't feel as though she was intruding.

Doing my best Sigmund Freud, I decided that the rack represented CF. I was hiding under it, afraid to venture out and explore the world or try anything new, though the mall was filled with great smells from the food court, cool clothes, music, and laughing couples. But I was scared of emerging from the "protection" of my ignorance about CF. Knowing too much about it might mean that I'd have to confront terrifying details, like my life expectancy. Books and doctors were often pessimistic. But this girl knew I didn't have to go it alone and she gently tried to pull me into the world while making sure I was O.K.

If I could get back into that dream, when I got to the part where she asked me, "Do you need any help?" instead of saying "No," I'd say, "Tell me who you are" or "What can you help me with?" I don't feel I can manipulate the dream, though I'm curious. And I'm not even certain the girl is Wendy. But hey, it's my dream. What it means is up to me. So I choose to believe the solicitous girl who appears every few years is my older sister, making a guest appearance in my subconscious to check up on her baby bro.

I decided it was time to return the favor and check up on her. So nearly three decades after she died, I decided to visit her grave. That was the easy part. Deciding what to do once I was at the cemetery was more difficult. The Jewish custom when you visit a grave is to place a small stone on it to show that you've been there. Because this would be my first visit and there was a lot to catch up on, I decided to write Wendy a letter telling her everything I wanted her to know.

I tucked it in my pocket and headed to the cemetery on a sunny Saturday morning. I assumed I'd be drawn to her grave, sister tugging brother to "That Spot." But once I got to the cemetery, there were so many grave-stones that I couldn't find Wendy at all.

I wandered around the cemetery for an hour hoping

my instinct would lead me to my baby sister's grave. It didn't. I had to ask for directions to "Babyland" – which sounds like it should be a store that sells diapers and playpens. Instead, it was a section of the cemetery up a little hill with modest gravestones reminding anyone who visited that some of the dead barely had a chance to live.

I took a deep breath of chilly spring air and began to look for my sister. Holmes*...Jefferson*...Lipman. Wendy Carol Lipman. Nothing more, but that was enough. I'd never seen the stone before, yet I knew when I saw it that it was something I'd been searching for my whole life, even before I knew it existed. I looked at the cropped grass on the plot in front of the marker and sunk to my knees to get as close as possible to her. I felt a little queasy. I took a deep breath and looked around – there was no one in sight – and read her this letter:

Dear Wendy:

I know that you know who I am. I just wanted to thank you for always looking after me. I guess because you check up on me so often, you probably want to know more about me.

I am 25 years old. I have dirty blond hair and blue eyes. I'm a spitting image of our father. I inherited his sense of humor as well. Speaking of Dad, I work with him as a purchasing manager in his company. You'd be really proud of him. The company is doing extremely well.

I went to college at the University of Georgia. I play all sports, including basketball, football, softball, and tennis. I work out a lot, and I am writing a book about cystic fibrosis. I assume you know that I have this disorder too, but I have been more fortunate than you in that I have been able to overcome much of it. Do I have you to thank? I bet I do.

Wendy, I won't let CF defeat me. My mission in the book I'm writing is to combat this disorder and tell other people it can be done. I'm sorry that you died, but I am happy that you will always be with me.

When I ask Mom about you, she talks and talks about how pretty you were and how she misses you all the time. She brings a stuffed animal and flowers to your grave every year on your birthday. I didn't know that you died from CF. Mom told me because I asked her while writing this book. I was shocked. Mom had a difficult time dealing with your death, but she will always love you.

Sometimes I ask myself, "Why did Wendy die, and why did I survive?" Now it doesn't matter because we are in this battle together. We can take care of your murderer. Let me do the writing, and you just help me with what to say. I realized several weeks ago that you were the one in my dream. I want to thank you for always offering me your sisterly advice. I know I have always refused your help because I claim to be fine without it. The truth is I do need it.

I have so many questions, not only about CF, but also about you. Do you watch over me? Was it your idea that I would wake up on my twenty-fifth birthday thinking I should write a book? Do I have CF because God thought I might be able to help myself and others beat it? What's heaven like? Do you hang out with our family and my dog, Howard? If you do, please give him a hug from me, tell him I love him, and I'll be thinking of him on his birthday.

I guess you're wondering why I'm here. Well, I'm not sure myself. I guess I just wanted to know where you lived. I feel like part of me is missing because I never met you. Mom and Dad still love you very much. Oh yeah, I have another sister, Emily, who doesn't have CF and is a great kid. Maybe one day you could tell her who you are.

This is the closest I've ever been to your body, but I believe your soul lives inside me. I love you Wendy. I'll see you in my dreams.

Love,
Your brother Andy

P.S. – CF's days of dominance are numbered.

When I finished, the cemetery was silent again except for the birds and the rustle of branches. I ran my fingers across Wendy's name on her gravestone. And as I did, I noticed a small wildflower next to the marker. It was reaching for the sun as if to prove that she was nurturing something beautiful and wanted to share it with me. Another gift from my sister, a wish from Wendy that I'd be comforted and see that strength could come from pain.

I walked slowly to the car, wondering why I wasn't crying. I realized that the overriding feeling I had was one of happiness. Why should I be crying? I'd finally met Wendy.

I felt she'd met me, too, and I felt more sure of it after talking to Aunt Susie on the phone one day at work. I told her about the cemetery visit and how comforting it was, as well as how disconcerting it was. Our conversation made me wrestle again with why anyone should die after just 16 days of life. Susie listened and then told me something she'd never shared before.

"Wendy's death was very hard on your mother," she said slowly. "She was crazy for a while after your sister died. Your survival healed her. You helped make your mother happy."

I thought about that and it gave me some solace. I thought to myself, "It probably makes Wendy happy to know that Mom is content now." I was turning that thought over in my head when a strange thing happened.

One of the temps in the office brought in a fax for me. I figured it was a message from a vendor so I wasn't in a hurry to read it, but the handwritten note on the bottom caught my eye. It said only, "Thank you, Wendy." I glanced at the top and realized the fax was for someone else at the company. For some reason, the temp had thought it was mine. For reasons she could never imagine, I knew that though it wasn't addressed to Andy Lipman, the message was meant just for me.

29

A WISH FOR WENDY

Fall 1999 – Age 26

Since that first visit, I've been back to the cemetery many times to sit by Wendy's grave. I go every month or six weeks, most often during tough times, like when I get in an argument with my girlfriend or when work seems overwhelming. I even paused there after a 0-4 softball game to pull myself together. I didn't have the dream anymore. It was as if by going to the cemetery I was getting the "help" that was offered in my sleep.

These visits weren't something I discussed with my parents. I suspected my mom would feel sad and mull over what was missing in my life that prompted me to visit a cemetery, and my dad would tell me I should just "get over it." I didn't know if my friends would understand either. People as a rule didn't spend a lot of time in cemeteries.

Some people might think it's morbid for a guy in his

20s to make the 25-minute drive to a graveyard to sit by the burial site of his older, infant sister. Honestly, I didn't think of it as a cemetery. It was just where Wendy happened to be and where she could best hear me. All the times I'd visited "Babyland," there had never been anyone else there, so it was a good place to think without interruptions or distractions. I would tell Wendy about the disappointments and frustrations in my life, but before too long I realized there's a lot to be thankful for, too, so I would tell her about the good stuff as well.

I didn't feel like she answered, really – that would be a little strange, I guess – but I did feel that she listened empathetically, which was all I wanted. Sometimes I'd see wildflowers growing nearby and I'd pick them and put them on her grave.

It was during such a visit to the cemetery that I was thinking about what I could do to remember Wendy and help obliterate our mutual enemy, CF. Bringing everyone to the cemetery to see her grave would have been meaningful for me, but it wouldn't have any critical impact on CF. Instead, I got the idea to organize a softball tournament called "A Wish for Wendy." The proceeds would go to the CF Foundation in her memory. For the first time, people wouldn't be afraid to say her name, and even those who'd never heard of her or didn't know much about CF would begin to associate her name with a positive effort – helping to find a cure for this disease – instead of remembering her as yet another of its undeserving victims.

When I told my parents about my idea, they didn't immediately volunteer to join the team. I understood that. They were concerned that between sports, working out, work, and spending time with my friends, I'd overextend myself. Too late, I told them. Been doing that for quite some time. They also wondered – as did I, though of course I'd never admit it – how I'd ever pull something like that off. Organizing a fundraising event was a massive undertaking, and I'd never done anything like it before.

Still, by now you know that I never let lack of experience or the threat of obstacles stop me. If that were the case, I'd never have tried out for any sports teams or gone to college or started working out. The more I'm told it can't be done, the more eager I am to do it. You know what they say: Don't be afraid to try something new. The ark was built by amateurs. The Titanic was built by experts.

To make "A Wish for Wendy" a success, I had to get some experienced people in my corner. That meant my mom, organizer and coordinator extraordinaire. She said she'd think about the "Wish for Wendy" idea. I thought maybe she wouldn't want to be involved, that it might be too hard on her. But that wasn't the case. She asked, "Can I help you? It's time we did something." I'm no dummy – I made her the volunteer coordinator. My dad helped, too, by sending letters soliciting support. He claims he didn't do much, but he got the ball rolling and people who might not have otherwise contributed sent checks. Even Emily pitched in. She raised hundreds of dollars on her own, which just astounded me.

My friends were amazing, too. They told their friends about the benefit, organized teams, and handled all the little details. To be honest, I didn't know how big this would be, and at first I worried that no one would be interested. But my friends proved me wrong.

We had 400 people playing ball at Piedmont Park, which was, you'll remember, the downtown Atlanta park where the Peachtree Road Race ended each year. I wanted to hold the CF benefit there because I associated the park with success and achieving one of the biggest goals of my life. It's a good thing I chose a large site because by day's end more than 500 people, including volunteers and players, took part in the softball tournament. We had a DJ, a local radio personality, and the Atlanta Falcon cheerleaders as well as lots of people who wanted to play ball and enjoy great food on a sunny fall day.

By now you know I can't share a story without having some mysterious "coincidence" or element that is personally significant and inexplicable. Here's one from the tournament: One team made the championship, but they were short a player, and it had to be a girl because the team was coed. If they didn't find someone to play in the championship game, they'd have to forfeit. They hunted around and finally found a player who agreed to join the team for that game. You can guess her name. Yup, Wendy. And I should tell you that they won the game by one run. True story!

Even after the tournament, donations kept coming in. When I closed the books in December, we'd raised nearly $30,000, all of it going to the CF Foundation. I felt really good about that, so good that I've decided that "A Wish For Wendy" won't be just a one-time thing. It's going to be an annual event until a cure for CF is found. That day will come, I promise, and I hope you'll work with me to make it happen sooner rather than later.

30

WORDS TO LIVE BY

Fall 2001 – Age 28

What a life I've lived! My parents were told I'd live 12 years. Later, I read that I'd be fortunate to be alive at 25. I almost ended my own life at 20. But I stand before you today, 28-years-old, an avid weightlifter, an author, and a leader.

My pulmonary function scores are at their highest. I'm lifting weights 4 to 5 times a week. This summer, I completed my fifth Peachtree Road Race. I'm still dating Andrea and our relationship couldn't be better. Recently, she gathered several of my friends to write letters to the 2002 Torch Relay Committee in Salt Lake City. And with their help, I was notified that I will be carrying the Olypmic torch on December 4, 2001. I have never been so excited in my life!

Bottom line: For now, CF remains incurable. But I learned that there's one thing that *can* defeat this killer:

attitude. It took me nearly 28 years to discover that the more positive I am, the better I feel. The more determined I am to feel better, the better I feel. Sure, there are things like infections I can't control. But rather than seeing them as doorways to my demise, I accept them for what they are – temporary setbacks, that's all. It's all about attitude.

The day I was born, my parents were told I'd be fortunate to see my teens. That same day, my Grandma Rose put me in her arms and looked deep into my blue eyes. After a few moments, she boldly predicted, "He's going to be a miracle. I just know it. He's a fighter." I can't say my grandmother was a psychic but her *attitude* changed everyone's outlook in that room. She was a fighter too – a survivor of the Holocaust.

I'd like to leave you with this thought: If you believe in yourself and work hard, you can accomplish many of your dreams. And if people belittle your dreams, telling you that you can't possibly bench-press 300 pounds, or graduate from a major university, or live past 25, ignore them. Ignore them and boldly follow each and every one of your dreams!

Seventeen years ago, when I was in sixth grade, a girl named Julie asked me if I was going to die. I didn't know how to respond. Now I finally have an answer: "Sure, I'm going to die – when I'm done living."

ACKNOWLEDGMENTS

*I want to thank Chiron Corporation
for their support of my book.*

*I want to thank June Bell and Michael Kanell
for their assistance with the original manuscript.*

*I want to thank my parents, my sister Emily,
and all my friends and family for their
support of this venture.*